THE ANATOMY OF THE HUMAN BODY

THE ANATOMY OF THE HUMAN BODY

BY

WILLIAM CHESELDEN

GYAN

ISBN : 978-81-212-1764-4(HB)

First Published, 1726

Published, 2018

Published by

Gyan Publishing House
5, Ansari Road
Daryaganj, New Delhi-110002
Phone: 011-47034999, 9811692060
www.gyanbooks.com
E-mail: books@gyanbooks.com

Printed at: G. Print Process, Delhi.

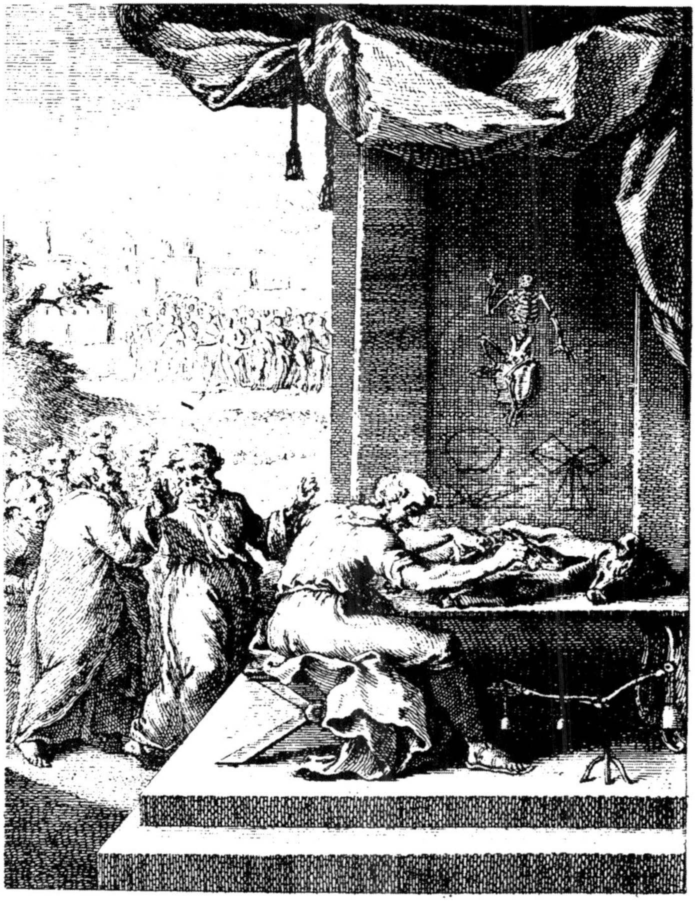

TO

Dr *Richard Mead*,

Physician to the KING,

FELLOW of the College of

Physicians in LONDON,

And of the

ROYAL SOCIETY.

SIR,

EVERY part of PHYSICK may justly presume on Your protection, to whom it owes so much improvement. ANATOMY in particular has received such advantage from Your LECTURES, that it were a kind of injustice not to dedicate all endeavours in that way to You; in me indeed it would be unpardonable not to offer the

a fruits

fruits of thoſe ſtudies, which at firſt began, and have ſtill been carried on with Your encouragement. The kind reception my induſtry has met with, is owing to You, the authority of whoſe opinion has in every place ſecured me ſo much favour; eſpecially in that ſeat of learning, which with diſtinguiſhed honours rewarded Your merit. I am,

SIR,

Your moſt obliged and

obedient humble Servant.

WILLIAM CHESELDEN.

PREFACE.

THE study of ANATOMY *as it leads to the knowledge of nature and the art of healing, needs not many tedious descriptions nor minute dissections; what is most worth knowing is soonest learn'd, and least the subject of disputes; while dividing and describing the parts, more than the knowledge of their uses requires, perplexes the learner, and makes the science dry and difficult.*

THIS edition is a tenth part larger than the former; not encreased by descriptions but by observations upon the uses and mechanism of the parts, with operations and cases in surgery.

THE plates are more in number, larger, better designed, and better executed than those which were in the former editions, which has unavoidably enhanced the price of this.

THE frontispiece represents the story of HIPPOCRATES *going to cure* DEMOCRATES *of madness; but finding him dissecting, to discover the seat of the Bile, he pronounced him the wisest man in* Abdera.

THE print in the title page represents a person drawing in a camera obscura, such a one as was used in this work.

CONTENTS.

BOOK. I.

BOOK II.

BOOK III.

BOOK IV.

Adver-

Advertiſement

SINCE the laſt edition of this book, I have publiſhed ſome Obſervations and caſes in ſurgery, with prints of operations and a ſet of chirurgical inſtruments. Theſe are annexed to a tranſlation of LE DRAN's Operations by Mr. GATAKER; and as ſome of them relate to my Anatomy, I thought it proper to take notice of them here: at the ſame time, in juſtice to the merit of Mr. LE DRAN, I would recommend a careful peruſal of his book to all practitioners in ſurgery.

W. CHESELDEN.

THE ANATOMY OF THE Human Body.

GENERAL INTRODUCTION.

IT is a received opinion, that an animal body is a compages of veſſels, variouſly diſpoſed, to form parts of different figures, for different uſes. The antients ſuppoſed that the heart and brain were firſt formed, and that the other parts proceeded from them, and that the membranes were derived from the dura mater, or pia mater of the brain. They diſtinguiſhed all the parts into ſpermatic and ſanguineous; the former of which they derived from the brain, and the latter from the heart; and frequently engaged in diſputes about the derivation of parts; with many other things of the like nature, conſequences of their hypotheſes. But the moderns, by the aſſiſtance of glaſſes, having made more accurate obſervations, conclude, that all the parts exiſt in miniature, from the firſt formation of the fœtus; and that their increaſe is only the extenſion and thickning of their veſſels, and that no part owes its exiſtence to another. Thus much I thought neceſſary to premiſe, that the reader might ſee for what reaſon no notice is taken, in this treatiſe, of ſome diſtinctions and diviſions of parts, uſed by ancient anatomiſts, and thoſe who have copied after them.

THE conſtituent parts of the animal body, are, fibres, membranes, arteries, veins, lymphæducts, nerves, glands, excretory veſſels, muſcles, tendons, ligaments, cartilages, and bones; to theſe may be added, the hair and nails.

FIBRES, as they appear to the naked eye, are ſimple threads of the minuteſt blood veſſels or nerves, or both.

MEMBRANES are compages of fibres, expanded to cover, or line, any other part.

ARTERIES are tubes that ariſe from the ventricles of the heart, and thence dividing into branches, diſtribute the blood to every part of the body.

VEINS are tubes to collect and return the blood from the extremities of the arteries to the heart.

LYMPHÆDUCTS are fine pellucid tubes, to carry lymph from all parts, eſpecially the glands, which they diſcharge into the larger veins, and into the vaſa lactea.

NERVES are faſciculi of cylindrical fibres, which

ariſe

arise from the medulla oblongata of the brain, and the medulla spinalis, and terminate in all the sensitive parts. They are the immediate organs of sensation.

A GLAND secretory, is composed of an artery, vein, lymphatic, excretory duct, and nerve. The use of glands is to secrete fluids from the blood for divers uses.

EXCRETORY VESSELS are either tubes from glands to convey the secreted fluids to their respective places; or vessels from the small guts, to carry the chyle to the blood vessels: these last are called vasa lactea.

MUSCLES are distinct portions of flesh, which, by contracting, perform the motions of the body.

TENDONS are the same fibres of which the muscles are composed; but more closely connected, that they may possess less space in a limb, and be inserted in less room into a bone.

LIGAMENTS are strong membranes, or bodies of fibres closely united, either to bind down the tendons, or give origin to the muscles, or tie together such bones as have motion.

CARTILAGES are hard, elastic bodies, smooth and insensible: Their use is to cover the ends of the bones that have motion, to prevent their attrition, &c.

BONES are firm parts, to sustain, and give shape to the body, &c.

INTRODUCTION
TO THE BONES.

THE uſe of the bones is to give ſhape and firmneſs to the body, to be levers for the muſcles to act upon, and to defend thoſe parts from external injuries that are of greateſt conſequence to be preſerved; as the brain, ſpinal marrow, heart, &c. Their fibres, when firſt formed like the ſhells and ſtones of fruits, are very ſoft, until by the addition of a matter, which is ſecreted into them, they grow by degrees to the hardneſs of a cartilage, and then perfect bone: But this change is neither made in a very ſhort time, nor begun in all the parts of the ſame bone at once. Flat bones, that have their fibres directed to all ſides, begin to oſſify in or near a middle point; but the cylindrical bones, and all others whoſe fibres are nearly parallel, begin about the middle of each fibre, and thence ſhoot forth to their extremities; not always in continued lines, but frequently beginning new oſſifications, which ſoon join the former; and by the continual addition of this oſſifying matter, the bones increaſe till their hardneſs reſiſts a farther extenſion; and their hardneſs always increaſing while they are growing, the increaſe of their growth becomes ſlower and ſlower, until they ceaſe to grow at all. In old and conſumptive perſons; and ſometimes in diſeaſed or wounded limbs, they decreaſe as well as the fleſhy parts, though not ſo faſt, becauſe of their hardneſs. Sometimes the oſſifying matter flows out of the bones, and forms bony excreſcences; and frequently in very old men it fixes on the arteries, and makes them grow bony; and when this happens to a degree, the arteries loſe their power to propel the blood, until the extreme parts mortify. And though the cartilages and arteries are moſt ſubject to theſe changes, yet no part is ſecure from them; for I have ſeen a large part of the muſcular fibres of the heart itſelf perfectly oſſified. I have known one inſtance of a deficiency of this oſſifying matter, in the lower jaw of an adult body; where all that part on one ſide, which is beyond the teeth, was of a ſubſtance between that of a cartilage and a ligament. In children that have died of the rickets, I have found the nodes on the bones ſoft, ſpongy, and bloody, and in one ſubject ſeveral of them as limber as leather, and the perioſtæum in ſome places many times its natural thickneſs; but the cartilages and cartilaginous epiphyſes had no apparent alteration in their texture, though ſome were ſwelled to more than twice their natural diameters.

Every cylindrical bone has a large middle cavity, which contains an oily marrow, and a great number of leſſer cells towards their extremities, which contain a bloody marrow. The bloody marrow is alſo found in all ſpongy cells of bones. The uſe of the firſt kind of marrow, I imagine, is to ſoften, and render leſs brittle, the harder fibres of bones near which it is ſeated; and that the other marrow is of the ſame uſe to the leſs compact fibres, which the more oily marrow might have made too ſoft; and that for this reaſon there is leſs of the oily marrow, and more of the bloody, in young bones than in old ones. Every one of theſe cells is lined with a fine membrane, and the marrow in the larger cells is alſo contained in thin membranous veſicles; in which membranes the veſſels are ſpread, which enter obliquely, about the middle of the cylindrical bones, from ſome of whoſe branches the marrow is ſecreted, while others of them enter the internal ſubſtance of the bones for their nouriſhment; and the reaſon why they enter obliquely is, that they may not weaken the bones by dividing too many fibres in the ſame place. If the bones had been formed of the ſame quantity of matter without any cavities, they would, if they were ſtreight, be able to ſuſtain the ſame weight: But being made hollow, their ſtrength to reſiſt breaking tranſverſely is encreaſed as much as their diameters are encreaſed, without encreaſing their weights; which mechaniſm being yet more convenient for birds, the bones of their wings, and for the ſame reaſon their quills, have very large cavities. But the bones in the legs of all animals are more ſolid, being formed to ſupport

port weight; and mens bodies being ſupported by two limbs, the bones of thoſe limbs are therefore made more ſolid than thoſe of quadrupeds. Inſects, and moſt of the ſmalleſt animals, have ſhells inſtead of bones, like lobſters, which ſerve them alſo for defence; and the muſcles, being inſerted into the ſhells at a greater diſtance from the center of motion of each joint than in animals that have bones, their motions are neceſſarily ſlower, ſtronger and more ſimple. Therefore in this ſort of animals, quickneſs of motion, where it is wanted, is procured by a number of joints, as may be ſeen in the legs of a flea; and variety of motions by joints with different directions, as may be obſerved in a lobſter. In a fractured bone, in which the ſame kind of matter that oſſified the bones at firſt is thrown out from the broken ends of a bone, there is formed a maſs of callous matter, of equal ſolidity with any part of the bone, and of equal or greater diameter, which will make the ſtrength of the bone in that place greater than it was before; which is very convenient; for bones, when broke, are ſeldom or never ſet in ſo good a direction as that in which they were firſt formed, and therefore they would be more liable to be broke in the ſame place again, and would be reunited with greater difficulty, and ſometimes not at all, becauſe the callus, being leſs vaſcular than a bone, it does not ſo eaſily admit the oſſific matter to flow through it to form a new callus.

Bones that are without motion, as thoſe of the ſcull, the oſſa innominata, &c. alſo bones with their epiphyſes, when they meet, preſs into each other, and form ſutures, which ſoon diſappear in thoſe that join, while their oſſific matter is ſoft; but thoſe that grow harder before they meet, preſs more rudely into each other, and make more uneven ſutures, ſome of which in the ſcull endure to the greateſt age: And ſometimes while a bone is oſſifying from its center, a diſtant part begins a new oſſification, and forms a diſtinct bone, which may happen to be of any figure. Theſe bones are ofteneſt found in the lambdoidal ſuture, and are there called oſſa triquetra. But the ends or ſides of bones that are intended for motion, are hindered from uniting, by the cartilages which cover them; for when theſe cartilages are eroded, the bones very readily unite, and form an anchyloſis.

The ends of all the bones that are articulated for very manifeſt motions, or that are not placed againſt other bones; are tipped with epiphyſes or additional bones; which in ſome meaſure determine their growth and figure; for if they had nothing to give bounds to them, they would ſhoot out like the callus from the broken ends of a bone that is ill ſet, and grow as ragged as the edges of bones which are joined by ſutures; and ſometimes epiphyſes are made uſe of to raiſe proceſſes upon bones for the inſertions of muſcles, as the trochanters of the thigh bones, where it would weaken the

the bones too much to have processes raised out of their substance.

The fibres of bones, for aught that we can discover from experiments or microscopical observations, appear to be connected to each other by the same means that the parts of a fibre are connected, that is, by the strong attraction which belongs to particles of matter in contact: but this cohesion of fibre to fibre is not equal to that in the parts of a fibre, though very nearly. Indeed if it was, a bone would not be a structure of fibres, but one uniform mass, like that of any pure metal, the cohesion of the parts of which are every where alike. Nor are the parts of bones disposed into visible lamellæ, stratum super stratum; as many have painted; for though young bones may in some places be split into lamellæ, yet they not only appear one solid uniform mass to the naked eye, but even with a microscope, till we come to their inner spongy texture, which also appears uniform. Their texture, when first formed, is every where loose and spongy; but as they increase, they become in many places very compact and dense, which results in great measure from the pressure of the bellies of the muscles, and other incumbent parts; as appears from the impressions they make on the surfaces of the bones, and the rough spines that rise on the bones in the interstices of the muscles, which are very remarkable in men who have been bred up in hard labour. In those parts of the flat bones that

that receive but little preſſure, the outer laminæ only become compact and denſe, while the middle part remains ſpongy; but where the preſſure is greater, as on the ſcapula and the middle of the ilium, they become, in an adult, one denſe body or table, and are uſually thinner in thoſe places than in a child before it is born. The cylindrical or round bones, being preſſed moſt in their middles, become there very hard and ſtrong, while their extremities remain ſpongy, and dilate into large heads, which make ſtronger joints, and give more room for the origins and inſertions of the muſcles; and increaſe the power of the muſcles, by removing their axis farther from the centre of motion of any joint they move.

All the bones, except ſo much of the teeth as are out of the ſockets, and thoſe parts of other bones, which are covered with cartilages, or where muſcles or ligaments ariſe or are inſerted, are covered with a fine membrane, which upon the ſcull is called pericranium, elſewhere periostæum. It ſerves for the muſcles to ſlide eaſy upon, and to hinder them from being lacerated by the roughneſs and hardneſs of the bones. It is every where full of ſmall blood veſſels, which enter the bones for their nouriſhment; but the internal ſubſtance of the larger bones is nouriſhed by the veſſels, which enter obliquely through their middles, as has been before obſerved.

CHAPTER

CHAPTER I.

Sutures and bones of the cranium.

A SUTURE is made by the mutual indentation of one bone with another. Thofe which have proper names are here defcribed; thofe which have not, derive their names from the bones they furround, and are known by them.

SUTURA CORONALIS runs acrofs the fcull, from one upper edge of the fphenoidal bone to the other, and joins the parietal bones to the frontal.

SUTURA SAGITTALIS joins the parietal bones; begins at the os occipitis, and is continued to the os frontis, in children down to the nofe; the os frontis in them being two bones, and fometimes fo in adult bodies.

SUTURA LAMBDOIDALIS joins the back part of the offa bregmatis, or parietal bones, to the upper part of the occipital: In this future are frequently obferved fmall bones called offa triquetra, and fometimes in other futures.

SUTURA SQUAMOSA is made by the upper part of the temporal and fphenoidal bones wrapping over the lower edges of the parietal bones.

SUTURA TRANSVERSALIS runs acrofs the face, through the bottoms of the orbits of the eyes; it joins the lower edge of the frontal bone to the os fphenoides, maxillæ fuperioris, offa nafi, ungues, plana, palati, and jugalia, or malarum.

THE

THE ſcull being divided into many bones, is neither ſo ſubject to fractures, nor to have fractures ſo far extended, as it would have been were it compoſed of one bone only. This ſtructure is alſo convenient for the oſſification of the bones, as has been already ſhewn, and for the birth; becauſe theſe bones not being perfect at that time, may be preſſed together, and make the head leſs.

TEN of the bones of the head compoſe the cranium, to contain the brain and defend it from external injuries.

OSSA PARIETALIA or BREGMATIS are two large bones which compoſe the ſuperior and lateral parts of the ſcull; on the inſide they are remarkably imprinted by the arteries of the dura mater.

OS FRONTIS makes the upper and fore part of the cranium; its lower parts compoſe the upper parts of the orbits of the eyes, where on its inſides are impreſſed the volvuli of the brain, which unevenneſſes help to keep that part of the brain ſteddy. In its middle above the os ethmoides uſually ariſes a thin ſpine, which ſtrengthens that part of the bone, it being otherwiſe weak from its flatneſs. In ſome ſculls this ſpine is wanting; but then the bone is uſually thicker in that place, and from its middle, externally, goes a proceſs which ſupports the bones of the noſe. Immediately above the os ethmoides in this bone is a ſmall blind hole, through which runs a vein into the beginning of the longitudinal ſinus of the dura mater; and on the upper edge

edge of each orbit, a ſmall perforation, or a notch, through which nerves and an artery paſs ſecure to the forehead; it has alſo a ſmall hole in each orbit, near the os planum, through which paſſes a branch of the fifth pair of nerves. In the ſubſtance of this bone near the noſe are two, three, four, and ſometimes five ſinuſes, which open into the noſe; they differ very much in different perſons, and are very rarely found in children. Theſe ſinuſes, and the ſpine in this bone, make it very dangerous, if not impracticable, to apply a trephine on the middle and lower part of the forehead.

Os ETHMOIDES, or CRIBRIFORME, is a ſmall bone, about two inches in circumference, ſeated in the anterior part of the baſis of the ſcull, being almoſt ſurrounded by the laſt deſcribed bone. It is full of holes, like a ſieve, through which, it is ſaid, the olfactory nerves paſs; which I could never diſcover. In its middle ariſes a large proceſs named chriſta galli: and oppoſite to this a thin one which in part divides the noſe. The greatet part of the laminæ ſpongioſæ in the noſe belong to this bone.

Os SPHENOIDES is of a very irregular figure; it is ſeated in the middle of the baſis of the ſcull, bounded by the os frontis, ethmoïdes, vomer, occipitis, maxillæ ſuperioris, oſſa parietalia, palati, malarum, temporum, and petroſa, which are parts of the former bones. In its inſide next the brain is a cavity named ſella turcica, which is bounded by four proceſſes called clinoides; under the two foremoſt

of

of which paſs the internal carotid arteries, and from their outſides are continued two thin long proceſſes upon that part of the frontal bone, which ſeparates the anterior lobes of the brain from the poſterior; oppoſite to the ſella turcica is a proceſs which makes part of the ſeptum narium. On the outſide of the ſcull adjoining to the upper jaw, are two proceſſes of this bone on each ſide, named pterygoides, from which ariſe one on each ſide near the palate, which have no name. Over theſe paſs the tendons of the pterygoſtaphylini externi muſcles; and nearer towards the occiput, between theſe and the ſtyloid proceſſes of the oſſa petroſa, ariſe two more ſmall rugged proceſſes; and under the ſella turcica, in this bone, is a ſinus or two, for the moſt part, in adults, but in children only ſuch a ſpongy ſubſtance as is ſeen in the ends of ſome of the bones. Dr. Nichols obſerves, this ſinus belongs properly to the os ethmoides. At the inſide of the baſis of the two anterior clinoid proceſſes are two round holes, which are the firſt foramina of the ſcull; through theſe the optic nerves paſs; almoſt under theſe, towards the ſides of the ſcull, are two irregular ſlits, named foramina lacera, or the ſecond foramina of the ſcull, through which paſs nerves and blood veſſels into the orbits of the eyes; and under theſe, towards the occiput, are two round holes, which are the third foramina, through which paſs nerves to the face; about half an inch nearer the occiput are two more, of an oval figure, which are the fourth fora-

foramina, through which paſs the largeſt branches of the fifth pair of nerves; and a ſtraw's breadth farther two very ſmall ones, called the fifth foramina, through which thoſe branches of the carotid arteries enter that are beſtowed upon the dura mater. Between this laſt deſcribed bone and the oſſa petroſa are two large rough holes, in which I have ſeen large veins; and from theſe holes, through part of the os ſphenoides, under the pterygoid proceſſes, are ſmall holes, through which paſs arteries to the back part of the noſe.

OSSA TEMPORUM are ſituated below the parietal bones, at the middle and lower parts of the ſides of the ſcull; they have each at their back parts one large ſpongy proceſs, called mammillaris, or maſtoideus; and from the lower and middle parts of each a proceſs which joins the oſſa malarum, named jugalis or zygomaticus.

OSSA PETROSA lie between the former bones and the occipital bones, or are truly portions of the former bones, being never found ſeparate in adult bodies. They have each on their outſides one long ſlender proceſs called ſtyliformis, and near the ſide of this proceſs a foramen, which runs obliquely forwards into the ſcull, through which the carotid arteries paſs to the brain; theſe are the ſixth foramina, and one foramen in the inſide of the ſcull leading to the organs of hearing, which are the ſeventh foramina. The ridge on the upper parts of each of theſe bones helps to keep the brain ſteddy, and are ſtrong ſupports to the thin and flat parts of the ſcull, which elſe would be exceeding weak. What remains of this bone belongs properly to a diſcourſe on the organs of hearing.

BETWEEN the laſt deſcribed bones and the following bone, are two large holes, which are the eighth foramina. Through theſe holes paſs the eighth pair of nerves and lateral ſinuſes; ſometimes they are two on each ſide, one for the nerve and one for the ſinus. To theſe we may add another very ſmall one on each ſide, through which paſs the portiones duræ of the auditory nerves; and ſometimes there is another for an artery.

OS OCCIPITIS makes all the back part of the ſcull: It is bounded by the ſphenoidal, temporal, petroſal, and parietal bones; it has two ſmall apophyſes, by which it is articulated to the ſpine; near thoſe apophyſes are two ſmall foramina, which are the ninth of the ſcull; through theſe paſs the ninth pair of nerves; and between theſe is the great or tenth foramen, through which the medulla oblongata deſcends into the ſpine, the cervical arteries enter, and the cervical veins paſs out. In the inſide of this bone is a crucial ſpine impreſſed by the longitudinal and lateral ſinuſes; and on the outſide, oppoſite to the middle of this ſpine, in ſome bodies, is an apophyſis, and from that down to the great foramen a ſmall thin ſpine. The ſpines in this bone are of the ſame uſe with thoſe in the os frontis, &c. viz. to ſtrengthen it. The thinner

parts

parts of this bone are alſo defended by the muſcles that cover them; which proviſion is very neceſſary, becauſe we can leaſt defend this part, and blows here are of worſe conſequence than on any other part of the ſcull, becauſe wounds in the cerebellum, which is underneath, are mortal. There are in moſt ſculls a foramen behind each apophyſis of the occipital bone; through which paſs ſinuſes from the lateral ſinuſes to the external cervical veins: By means of theſe communications, as in all other communications of the ſinuſes, the blood paſſes from thoſe that happen to be ſurcharged by any poſture of the head, into thoſe that from the ſame poſture would have been almoſt empty. Such ſculls as want theſe foramina have two ſinuſes for the ſame purpoſe.

CHAPTER II.

Of the bones of the face, &c.

OSSA NASI make the upper part of the noſe; they form that kind of arch which is fitteſt to ſuſtain ſuch injuries as the noſe is moſt expoſed to.

OSSA MALARUM. Theſe bones compoſe the anterior, lower, and outer parts of the orbits of the eyes; they have each a ſhort proceſs, which proceſſes join the proceſſus jugales of the temporal bones, and form arches which have been called oſſa jugalia.

Ossa ungues are ſeated immediately below the os frontis towards the noſe in the orbits of the eyes; whoſe anterior and inner parts they help to compoſe; and between each of them and the upper jaw is a foramen as large as a gooſe quill, into which the puncta lacrymalia lead, to carry off any ſuperfluous moiſture from the eyes into the noſe.

Ossa plana are ſeated immediately beyond the foregoing bones, in the orbits of the eyes, and are near thrice as big. They are rather ſmooth ſurfaces of the os ſpongioſum, than diſtinct bones, and are very often imperfect.

Maxilla superior is always deſcribed ſingle, though it is manifeſtly divided by a ſuture which is ſcarce ever obliterated; it has two proceſſes, which join the os frontis, and make part of the noſe; and another, which joins to the cartilage of the ſeptum naſi. Its upper and outward parts make the lower parts of the orbits of the eyes; its lower ſide, all that part of the face under the cheeks, eyes, and noſe to the mouth, and two thirds of the roof of the mouth. A little below the orbits of the eyes, in this bone, are two holes, and behind the dentes inciſores one more, which divides into two, as it opens into the noſe, on each ſide the ſeptum naſi. Between the poſterior grinding-teeth and the orbits of the eyes are two great ſinuſes, called antra maxillæ ſuperioris, which open into the upper part of the

the noſe. And in the lower edge of this jaw are the alveoli, or ſockets for the teeth. Part of the ſides of theſe cavities, that lie next the noſe, are only membranes which make the cavities like drums, perhaps to give a grave ſound to the voice when we let part of it through the noſe; but brutes not needing ſuch variety of ſounds, have theſe cavities open to the noſe, and filled with lamellæ, which are covered with membranes, in which the olfactory nerves terminate, for a more exquiſite ſenſe of ſmelling than is neceſſary for men. Impoſthumations ſometimes happen in theſe cavities: The ſigns of this diſeaſe are, great pain about the part, matter in the noſe on the ſide diſeaſed, ſtinking breath, and rotten teeth. Mr. COWPER firſt deſcribed this caſe, and the cure; which is performed by drawing out the laſt tooth but one, or two, or more if rotten; and through their ſockets making a perforation into the antrum; or if drawing a tooth makes a perforation, which ſometimes happens, and perhaps gave the firſt hint of this cure, then that opening muſt be enlarged, if it is not ſufficient to diſcharge the matter.

OSSA PALATI are two ſmall bones that make the back part of the roof of the mouth, and a ſmall part of the bottom of each orbit. Between the oſſa palati and os maxillare near the pterygoid proceſſes of the ſphenoidal bone, are two ſmall foramina, thro' which arteries and nerves paſs to the palate.

Os VOMER is ſeated between the bones of the palate, and the ſphenoidal bone. It is alſo joined to the proceſs of the ethmoides, and part of the lower jaw. Its fore part is ſpongy, and is continued to the middle cartilage of the noſe. This bone and cartilage are the ſeptum naſi.

Os SPONGIOSUM is uſually treated as a diſtinct bone, though it is only the ſpongy laminæ in the noſe, of the os ethmoides and oſſa plana, but chiefly of the os ethmoides, to which it always adheres. In conſidering theſe lamellæ as a diſtinct bone, we follow the ancients, who did not diſtinguiſh the bones of the ſcull only, as they are divided by ſutures, but according to the differences of their texture, figure, ſituation, or uſe. Thus they called theſe parts os ſpongioſum; a proceſs of the temporal bone, joined to the os malæ, os jugale, &c.

MAXILLA INFERIOR is articulated with looſe cartilages to the temporal bones, by two proceſſes, named condyloides. Near theſe ariſe two more, called coronales, and at the inſide of the chin a ſmall rough proceſſus innominatus. In the inſide of this bone, under each proceſſus coronalis, is a large foramen, which runs under the teeth, and paſſes out near the chin. In this foramen, the veſſels paſs that belong to the teeth; and in the upper edge of this jaw are the ſockets for the teeth, which ſeldom exceed ſixteen in each jaw; the four firſt in each are called inciſores, the two next canini, the reſt molares; the four laſt of theſe are named dentes

dentes ſapientiæ, becauſe they do not appear till men arrive at years of diſcretion. The inciſores and canini have only one ſingle root, but the molares more; the eight firſt, two; and the reſt, ſome three, ſome four, eſpecially in the upper jaw; where alſo they are ſpread wider, becauſe that jaw being more ſpongy than the other, the teeth need more ſpace to fix them. Each of theſe roots has a foramen, through which paſs an artery, vein, and nerve, which are expanded in a fine membrane that lines the cavity in each tooth. Theſe veſſels and membrane are the ſeat of the tooth-ach. The teeth of children caſt off while they are growing; but the ſucceeding teeth ariſe in new ſockets, deeper and larger than the former, for the jaws increaſing faſter than the teeth, muſt otherwiſe have left chaſms between them, ſuch as are in the mouths of brutes; but where teeth are drawn in adult bodies, the ſockets cloſe, and new ones very rarely ſucceed.

CHAPTER III.

Of the bones of the trunk.

THE bones of the trunk are thoſe which compoſe the ſpine or chain of bones from the head down to the rump, the ribs and ſternum, to which may juſtly be added the oſſa innominata.

THE ſpine is compoſed of twenty four vertebræ

(each of which in a young child is three bones) besides those of the os sacrum and coccygis; seven belong to the neck, the first of which is called atlas, because it immediately supports the head; its upper side has two cavities, into which the apophyses of the os occipitis are received; but these two cavities together, unlike all other joints, are laterally portions of concentric circles, by which means they are but as one joint, and so suffer the head to move easily side-ways, which otherwise it could no more do than the knee, which also has two heads and two cavities. The under side of this bone has a very flat articulation with the next, which fits it for a rotatory motion. The second vertebra is called dentata, or axis, from a process which passes thro' the former bone, and is the axis upon which it turns; nevertheless all the vertebræ of the neck contribute something to the rotatory motion of the head. The processus dentatus is strongly tied to the os occipitis, and to the atlas by ligaments, to prevent its hurting the spinal marrow. Twelve of which belong to the back, five to the loins. The os sacrum is sometimes five, sometimes six bones, and the os coccygis four. If this chain had been composed of fewer bones, they must have either not been capable of bending so much as they do, or have bent more in each joint, which would have pressed the spinal marrow, the ill consequences of which are sufficiently seen in persons grown crooked, or who have had distortions from external accidents.

THE

The uppermoſt vertebra of the neck being fixed behind the center of gravity of the head, the neck is therefore ſo far bent forward, as that the laſt of theſe vertebræ (which has a firm bearing upon thoſe of the thorax) may be exactly under the center of gravity. Thoſe of the thorax are bent backwards, behind the center of motion, to make room for the parts contained in the thorax; and, that they might not be made too weak by this ſtructure, they are formed for leſs motion than other vertebræ; and thoſe in particular, which are bent fartheſt from the center of gravity have the leaſt motion. The middle vertebræ of the loins are again bent forwards under the center of gravity, or near it; and from thence they go backwards to the os ſacrum, where being fixed to the oſſa innominata behind the center of gravity, the articulation is therefore firm and without motion, and from thence the oſſa innominata are ſo formed, as that their ſockets, into which the thigh bones are fixed, where there is a free motion, are exactly under the center of gravity. In brutes the ſpine is differently formed, according to the actions for which they are deſigned.

In all theſe vertebræ, except the firſt, is a middle anterior ſpongy body, by which they are firmly articulated with a very ſtrong intervening ligament; and from the middle of the hind part of each, except the firſt, ſtands a proceſs named ſpinalis, and from every one a proceſs on each ſide, called tranſverſalis, and two ſuperior, and two inferior ſhort ones; by which the back parts of the vertebræ are articulated, named obliqui, ſuperiores, and inferiores.

THE fore part of the ſeven vertebræ of the neck, and two upper of the back, are flat forwards, to make room for the aſpera arteria and gula: The third and fourth of the back acute, to give way to the veſſels of the lungs and heart, and bent to the right ſide for the better ſituation of the heart, which makes that ſide of the breaſt more convex than the other, and therefore ſtronger; which ſeems advantageous to the right arm, its motions depending upon the ſupport it receives from the breaſt. Hence, I think, it ſeems, that the almoſt univerſal preference of that arm is not an arbitrary thing, but founded upon obſervation, that it is capable of more perfect actions than the other.

THE ſpinal proceſſes of the ſecond, third, fourth, and fifth vertebræ of the neck are forked, the two laſt long and horizontal, the three or four upper ones of the back like them, only a little declining, the middle ones of the back run obliquely downwards, and the proceſſes of the remaining vertebræ become ſucceſſively thicker, ſtronger, and leſs declining; thoſe of the loins being horizontal, like the laſt of the neck. The muſcles, that are inſerted into the ſpinal proceſſes of the vertebræ of the neck and loins, will act with more ſtrength than thoſe of the

the back, becauſe their proceſſes being perpendicular to the ſpine, they are longer leavers: beſides, thoſe of the back almoſt touch one another, to prevent much motion, becauſe it would interrupt reſpiration; but more motion being neceſſary in the neck and loins, their proceſſes are made fit for it.

THE tranſverſe proceſſes of the vertebræ of the neck are perforated, for the admiſſion of the cervical blood veſſels, and bowed downwards, and hollowed, for the paſſage of the cervical nerves. The eight or nine upper ones of the back receive the upper ribs; and the reſt, with thoſe of the loins, ſerve only for origins and inſertions of muſcles.

OS SACRUM has two upper oblique proceſſes, ſome ſmall ſpinal proceſſes, and two foramina in each interſtice of the bones it is compoſed of, both before and behind. Oſſa coccygis have none of theſe parts.

THROUGH every bone of the ſpine, the oſſa coccygis excepted, is a large foramen, which together make a channel through the ſpine, in which is contained the medulla ſpinalis; and in each ſpace between the vertebræ are two large holes for the nerves to paſs out.

'TIS worth conſidering the proviſion which is made to prevent luxations in this chain of bones, ſuch luxations being worſe than any other, becauſe of the ſpinal marrow which is contained within theſe bones. The bodies of the vertebræ are all in the ſame

ſame manner connected by ſtrong intervening ligaments or cartilages. In the neck the oblique proceſſes of the received bone are wrapped over thoſe of the receiving bone, which forbids their luxating forwards. The tranſverſe proceſſes, with a ſmall apophyſis of the body of the ſame bone, in like manner, ſecure them from ſlipping backwards; and an apophyſis on each ſide of the body of the receiving bone, hinders them from ſlipping to either ſide. The vertebræ of the back are hindred from diſlocating forwards by the ſame proviſion with thoſe of the neck; and from luxating backwards, by the ribs which are faſtened to the tranſverſe proceſſes of the inferior vertebræ, and againſt the back part of the body of the next ſuperior: they alſo hinder them from diſlocating to either ſide; but the laſt ribs are not fixed to the tranſverſe proceſſes of the vertebræ of the back, and therefore it is that luxations are moſt frequently ſeen in this part; but the vertebræ of the loins are received into deep cavities, and are tied with much ſtronger ligaments for their ſecurity. Each joint of the vertebræ, except the two uppermoſt, has two centers of motion, one upon the bodies of the vertebræ, when the trunk is bowed forward; and the other at the articulations of the oblique proceſſes, when the body is bowed backwards; from which ſtructure the extenſors will have about twice the leaver to act with, and conſequently twice the power to raiſe the trunk into an erect poſture, that they have to carry it beyond that posture; for then the oblique processes begin to be the centre of motion, and give a like advantage to the benders. Without this contrivance it would be more difficult to keep the body erect, or to recover an erect posture with considerable strength after a bend of the body.

The ribs are twelve in number on each side; the seven uppermost are called true ribs, because their cartilages reach the sternum; and the five lowest are called bastard ribs. They are articulated to the bodies of the twelve vertebræ of the back, and all, except the two or three last, are articulated to their transverse processes, and the under side of the middle ribs are hollowed for the passage of the intercostal vessels. They defend the parts contained in the breast, and when they are drawn upwards, the cavity of the breast is enlarged for inspiration, and so the contrary. In two children, which I have dissected, I found the ribs broke inwards, and on the outside a very plain print of a thumb and fingers, occasioned by their nurses taking hold of their breasts, and hoisting them up on one hand, which being often repeated, had broke the ribs inwards like a green stick, without separating the broken ends of them. I have also very frequently seen the shape of childrens breasts quite spoiled by such tricks, which have occasioned weakness of body, crookedness, and other diseases.

Sternum, or breast-bone, is generally made up of three spongy bones, sometimes more; to this

the

the true ribs are articulated by their cartilages, which ſometimes in robuſt men have moveable joints, ſuch as are ſeen in oxen and other quadrupeds. At the end of the ſternum is the cartilago enſiformis, ſo called from its ſhape, but it very often is double; there is alſo frequently found variety in the form of the cartilages, which join the ribs and ſternum, ſometimes one cartilage ſerving two ribs, and ſometimes a cartilage not joined to any rib; frequently in old perſons we find parts of them oſſified, and I have twice found them totally oſſified in men between forty and fifty years of age, both of which died with a great difficulty of breathing; and beſides, one had a jaundice, and the other a dropſy, but the lungs in both were very ſound.

There are ſeldom found fewer than four and twenty vertebræ in the ſpine, beſides the os ſacrum, but often more; ſometimes thirteen of the back, with as many ribs of a ſide; and ſometimes ſix in the loins: and in ſome bodies two ribs from the firſt vertebra of the loins, but then it has wanted tranſverſe proceſſes.

Os innominatum is in young perſons compoſed of three bones; the upper is named ilium, the lower and poſterior os iſchii, and the anterior os pubis: the upper edge of the ilium is called its ſpine, the anterior part of the ſpine its apex, and a little lower is the proceſſus innominatus. Ilium has two proceſſes, the one named the obtuſe proceſs, and the other the acute; in the centre of

theſe

thefe bones is the acetabulum or focket for the thigh bone; in the bottom of which focket is another cavity, in which lies the lubricating gland of this joint. When impoftumations happen in this joint they ufually caufe a great fwelling and lamenefs in the hip, which, in time, makes a collection of matter in the external part of the hip; however, this is not the only way it proceeds, for I have twice feen the matter in the joint make way thro' the bottom of the acetabulum into the pelvis of the abdomen; in thefe cafes, when the patient went to ftool, the matter, by ftraining, was preffed out thro' the external wound.

CHAPTER IV.

Bones of the upper limb.

CLAVICULA is connected at one end to the fternum with a loofe cartilage, and at the other to the proceffus acromion of the fcapula; its chief ufe is to keep the fcapula a fufficient diftance from the breaft, by which means the fhoulders are hindered from coming near together, as they do in thofe quadrupeds which ufe their fore limbs only to walk on, and not as men do their hands.

SCAPULA is fixed to the fternum by the clavicula, but its chief connection is to the ribs and fpine, by thofe mufcles which are made alfo for its various

various motions; and in ſuch quadrupeds as have no clavicles it is fixed only by muſcles, whoſe actions give to this bone a great deal of that motion which ſeems to be in the joint of the ſhoulder. The under ſide of this bone is a little concave, partly to fit it to the outer ſurface of the ribs on which it moves, and partly to give room for the ſub-ſcapularis muſcle. On the outſide ariſes a large ſpine; the fore part of which is called the proceſſus acromion, to which the clavicula is fixed. In men and ſuch quadrupeds as have clavicles, and uſe their fore limbs like arms, this proceſs and ſpine are much larger and more prominent, not only for the better fixing the clavicle, but alſo to remove the muſcles farther from the center of motion, whereby they are able to move a greater weight. Near this proceſs is another called coracoides, from whoſe extremity, with like advantage, ariſe two muſcles of the arm; this proceſs with the former, and a flat ligament between them both, hinder the os humeri from being diſlocated upwards. The ſide oppoſite to the ſocket is called the baſis of the ſcapula, and the lower edge coſta inferior from its figure, which is thick, and like a rib to the ſcapula; but its upper edge being very thin, is improperly ſo called in the human ſceleton, though not ſo in many quadrupeds. At the fore part of this edge, cloſe to the coracoid proceſs, is a ſemicircular nitch for the paſſage of blood veſſels, which nitch is join-

ed

ed at top with a ligament, and ſometimes with bone.

Os HUMERI: its upper end or head, where it is joined to the ſcapula, is ſomewhat flat, and much larger than the ſocket which receives it. At the upper part are two proceſſes for the inſertions of muſcles of the arms; between theſe proceſſes is a long channel, in which lies a tendon of the biceps cubiti. At the lower end are two conſiderable proceſſes, both formed to give origins to muſcles of the wriſt and fingers; and the flexors of theſe joints being much more conſiderable than the extenſors, the inner proceſs from which the flexors ariſe is therefore much larger than the outer, from which the extenſors take their origin: between theſe proceſſes is the joint. That part to which the upper end of the radius is fixed, is fitted not only for the motion of the elbow, but alſo for the rotatory motion of the radius; the reſt of this joint is made of portions of unequal, but concentric, circles, like the ſhanks of quadrupeds; which inequality prevents the ulna from diſlocating ſideways, which ſo ſmall a joint with ſo much motion would be very ſubject to. Of a like uſe is the little ſinus on the fore part of the humerus, and the large one behind; the firſt of which receives a proceſs of the ulna when the arm is bent, and the other, the olecranon, when the arm is extended.

ULNA: at the upper end it has one large proceſs called olecranon, and a ſmall proceſs on the

fore

fore part; and on one ſide between theſe is alſo a ſmall cavity, which receives the upper end of the radius for its rotatory motion; and down the ſide of this bone, next the radius, is a ſharp edge, from which the ligament ariſes, which connects theſe bones together. At the lower end is a proceſs, called ſtyliformis, and a round head, which is received into the radius for the rotatory motion of the cubit.

Radius: its upper end is received into the ulna, and joined to the humerus, in a manner chiefly fitted for its rotatory motion, for the ſtrength of the elbow joint receives but little advantage from the union of theſe two bones. A little below this head is a large tubercle, into which the biceps muſcle is inſerted, which by the advantage of this inſertion turns the cubit ſupine, as well as bends it. At the lower end, which is thicker, is a ſocket to receive the carpus, and at the ſide next the ulna a ſmall one to receive that bone, and a thin edge, into which the tranſverſe ligament, which ariſes from the ulna, is inſerted. This ligament ties theſe bones conveniently and firmly together; for the ulna being chiefly articulated to the os humeri, and the radius to the carpus, a weight at the hand, without this ligament, would be liable to pull theſe bones aſunder.

Of the bones of the hand: Carpus is compoſed of eight bones of very irregular forms, undoubtedly the propereſt that can be; yet why in theſe forms

forms, rather than any other, no one has been able to ſhew. They have all obſcure motions one with another, and with thoſe of the metacarpus; but the motion of thoſe of the firſt rank, or order, with thoſe of the ſecond is more conſiderable, and are moved by the ſame muſcles which move the carpus on the radius. The metacarpus conſiſts of four bones which ſuſtain the fingers; that of the fore-finger having the leaſt motion, and that of the little one the moſt: the other ends of theſe bones have round heads for the articulations of the fingers; but the other joints of the fingers double heads and ſockets. The thumb is ſhorter and ſtronger than any of the fingers, becauſe in its actions it is to reſiſt them all. The firſt joint is very ſingular, each bone receiving and being equally received. The bones of the fingers on the inſide are flat and a little hollow, which is neceſſary to make room for the flexors of the fingers, and to render their ſhape proper for graſping; but this leſſening their diameters, and conſequently weakening them in the direction in which they are moſt liable to be broke, ſuch inconvenience is provided againſt by a larger ſubſtance.

CHAPTER V.

Bones of the lower limb.

OS FEMORIS at its upper end has a round head which is received into the ſocket of the os innominatum. In moſt quadrupeds this head is oblong, and makes a firmer articulation; but that ſhape will not allow of ſo much motion as a rounder head. The two proceſſes near the head are called the greater and leſſer trochanters, which are evidently formed for the inſertion of muſcles, as the neck which lies between theſe and the head, is formed to make room for that neceſſary quantity of muſcles which are ſeated on the inſide of the thigh, and alſo by projecting outwards to make long levers for the muſcles, which are inſerted into its upper and external parts. Between the great trochanter and the neck is a large ſinus, into which muſcles are inſerted: between the two trochanters is a remarkable roughneſs for the ſame uſe, from which begins the linea aſpera. The middle of this bone, for the conveniency of the muſcles, is bent forwards, which would make it ſubject to break backwards, if there was not a ſtrong ridge on the back ſide, which ſtrengthens it ſufficiently, and ſerves alſo for advantageous inſertions for ſeveral muſcles; this ridge is called the linea aſpera. At the lower end of this bone are two large heads, called the outer and

and inner apophyſes: theſe are ſo contrived, partly from being projected backwards, and partly from their ſhapes, as to remove the center of motion very far behind the axis of the bone, which gives great power to the muſcles that extend this joint to raiſe the whole weight of the body, though it leſſens the power of the benders which move the leg only; between theſe proceſſes the large veſſels deſcend ſecurely to the leg.

PATELLA is ſeated on the forepart of the knee; its firſt appearance is in the centre of the tendon, through which it ſoon extends, until the tendinous fibres are loſt, and appear to be converted into bone; however, when this bone is broke, the original tendinous fibres ſeem to prevail, ſeeing the broken parts, unlike all other bones when fractured, unite with a tendon-like ſubſtance, which is rarely converted into bone, and eſpecially in thoſe caſes where the joint recovers with moſt motion: its uſe is to ſecure the extenſors of the tibia, leſt paſſing over the joint, they might be too much expoſed to external injuries; it alſo increaſes the advantage (mentioned in the laſt paragraph) of removing the common axis of the extenſors of the tibia farther from the centre of motion, and is a moſt convenient medium for thoſe muſcles to unite in, to perform one common action.

TIBIA, the ſhin bone, is large at its upper end, where are two ſhallow ſockets which receive the thigh bone; between theſe is a rough proceſs, to which the crofs ligaments of this joint are connected. Near the upper end is a procefs, into which the ligament or tendon of the patella is inferted, and at the lower end is the procefs, which makes the inner ancle, and fecures this bone from diflocating outwards. Towards the upper end this bone is triangular, and even concave on the fide next the mufcles to make room for them; but lower, as the mufcles grow lefs and tendinous, the bone grows rounder; that being upon the whole a ftronger form; yet it is not made fo ftrong as the thigh bone, though it bears a greater weight, which it is able to do by being ftraighter, fhorter, and bearing the weight of the body in a more perpendicular direction.

Fibula is feated on the outfide of the tibia; its upper end is joined to that bone below the joint of the knee, and its lower end is received into a fhallow finus of the fame bone, and below that makes the external ancle; which procefs, with the procefs of the tibia, ftrengthens the ancle joint, which neverthelefs, being fo fmall, would have been not ftrong enough, if it had been made for more motion. It is doubtful to me, whether or not this bone contributes to the fupport of the body; but its great ufe is for the origins of mufcles, and even its fhape is fuited to theirs.

Of the bones of the foot: Tarfus is compofed of feven bones, the firft of which, called aftragalus, fupports the tibia, and is fupported by the os calcis,

calcis, which being projected backwards, makes a long lever for the muſcles to act with, that extend the ancle and raiſe the body upon the toes. Theſe two bones have a conſiderable motion between themſelves, and the aſtragalus alſo with the os naviculare, and all the reſt an obſcure motion one with another, and with the bones of the metatarſus, the greateſt part of theſe motions being towards the great toe, where is the greateſt ſtreſs of action: theſe bones thus giving way are leſs liable to be broke, and, as a ſpring under the leg, make the motion of the body in walking more eaſy and graceful, and the bones which are ſupported by them leſs ſubject to be fractured in violent actions. To theſe join five others, called the metatarſal bones; that which ſupports the great toe is much the largeſt, there being the greateſt ſtreſs in walking; under the end of this lie the two ſeſamoid bones, which are of the ſame uſe as the patella; the great toe has two bones, the leſſer three each, the two laſt of the leaſt toes frequently grow together.

CHILDREN are ſometimes born with their feet turned inwards, ſo that the bottom of the foot is upwards: in this caſe the bones of the tarſus, like the vertebræ of the back in crooked perſons, are faſhioned to the deformity. The firſt knowledge had of a cure of this diſeaſe was from Mr. PRESGROVE, a profeſſed bone-ſetter, then living in Weſtminſter. I recommended the patient to him, not knowing how to cure him myſelf. His way was by holding the foot as near the natural poſture as he could, and then rolling it up with ſtraps of ſticking plaſter, which he repeated from time to time, as he ſaw occaſion, until the limb was reſtored to a natural poſition, but not without ſome imperfection, the bandage waſting the leg, and making the top of the foot ſwell and grow larger. After this, having another caſe of this kind under my care, I thought of a much better bandage, which I had learnt from Mr. COWPER, a bone-ſetter at Leiceſter, who ſet and cured a fracture of my own cubit when I was a boy at ſchool. His way was, after putting the limb in a proper poſture, to wrap it up in rags dipped in the whites of eggs, and a little wheat flower mixed; this drying, grew ſtiff, and kept the limb in a good poſture. And I think there is no way better than this in fractures, for it preſerves the poſition of the limb without ſtrict bandage, which is the common cauſe of miſchief in fractures. When I uſed this method to the crooked foot, I wrapt up the limb almoſt from the knee to the toes, and cauſed the limb to be held in the beſt poſture 'till the bandage grew ſtiff, and repeated the bandage once a fortnight.

THE bones are ſubject to diſeaſes from all the ſame cauſes that the other parts are, but either from their hardneſs, inſenſibility, or other cauſes, they neither are ſo frequently diſeaſed, nor do their diſeaſes appear ſo various; and it is generally of more conſequence what texture the diſeaſed bone, or part of the bone is of, than from what cauſe that diſeaſe proceeded; for when diſeaſes happen upon the ſurfaces of the hard bones, they uſually admit a cure by exfoliation; but when matter is made in the ſpongy ends of the cylindrical bones, or in the bodies of other ſpongy bones, the matter, whatever was the firſt cauſe, inſinuates itſelf through thoſe ſpongy cells, ſwelling the bone, and making generally an incurable caries; but if the matter is corroſive, it often ulcerates theſe parts, and uſually makes ſo large a diſcharge as to deſtroy the patient where the part diſeaſed cannot be extirpated, which is often the caſe when matter is made in the bones in ſcrophulous habits.

THE venereal diſeaſe rarely attacks any but the hardeſt parts of the bones, very ſoon raiſing large tumors and caries or mortification; but theſe carious parts of bones from this or other cauſes are but partially mortified; for, were they perfectly ſo, the ſound and unſound parts would ſeparate, though the integuments were not taken off; whence it happens, that, where there is a good habit of body, carious bones are often endured many years without much inconvenience; and we find from experience, that ſuch ſeparations are not to be made till the diſeaſed part is laid bare and perfectly mortified, by being expoſed to the air, &c. and then the ſound part underneath ſeparating from the unſound, there firſt granulates a fungous fleſh-like appearance, which ought never to be treated with corroſive medicines, it conſtantly ſhrinking and hardening of itſelf, being the ſame ſubſtance which ſhoots from the ends of broken bones, where alſo it ſoon ſhrinks and converts into a callus to reunite them.

THERE is a caries diſtinct from theſe, which I have only ſeen in two patients who died after a long rheumatic diſorder, in which the outer ſurface of all the hardeſt bones, as the middle of the cylindrical bones, and the top of the ſcull, in one which I boiled, and in the other as far as I was allowed to examine, I found the outer part every where crumbly or ſcaly, falling into pieces like duſt or ſand, with very little appearance of tumor any where, and no appearance of diſeaſe in the ſpongy parts.

SOMETIMES matter is formed in the large medullary cavities of the cylindrical bones, which conſtantly increaſing and wanting vent, partly by corroding and rendering the bone carious, and partly by preſſure, tear aſunder the ſtrongeſt bone in an human body, of which I have known ſeveral inſtances. In one caſe, where the matter had ſufficient diſcharge by an external caries formed together with the internal one, all the internal hard part of the bone which contains the medulla was ſeparated from the reſt, and being drawn out through the place where the external caries made a vent, the patient received a perfect cure. In another caſe of this kind, where the internal part which contains the medulla was alſo ſeparated from the reſt, and there being

being holes through which the matter was difcharged, but none fufficient to take out the exfoliated bone; the matter continued to flow in great quantity till it deftroyed the patient; and poffibly if this cafe had been rightly known, the internal exfoliated part might have been taken out, and the patient cured. In both thefe cafes, it feems as if only fo much of the internal part of the bone was become carious, as receives nourifhment from the artery which enters the middle of the bone; and as a caries is a mortification of a bone, might not this difeafe arife from a hurt in the veffel which nourifhes that particular part?

CHAPTER VI.

Cartilages, ligaments, &c.

EVERY part of a bone which is articulated to another bone for motion, is covered or lined with a cartilage, as far as it moves upon, or is moved upon by another bone in any action; for cartilage being fmoother and fofter than bone, it renders the motions more eafy than they would have been, and prevents the bones wearing each other in their actions.

IN each articulation of the lower jaw, there is a loofe cartilage, upon which the condyloid procefs moves on one fide, while the jaw is moved to the other;

other; and the two processes being thus raised at once, the jaw is thrust forward. These cartilages are also found in animals that chew the cud, but not in beasts of prey, as far as I have examined, their articulations being also deeper and firmer; and in the otter particularly, sections of the sockets, which receive the condyloid processes of the lower jaw, are more than half circles; so that the jaw cannot be dislocated directly without breaking the sockets. This structure renders the motions of the jaw more firm, as that with intervening cartilages makes it more loose and voluble. There are also cartilages of this kind between the clavicles and the sternum.

In the joint of the knee are two loose, almost annular cartilages, which being thick at their outer edges, and thin at their inner ones, they make the greatest parts of the two sockets in this joint. The use of these cartilages is to make variable sockets to suit the different parts of the lower end of the os femoris; for none but a round head and a round cavity can suit in motion, unless the shape of one or the other alters; and it is plainly necessary, that this lower end of the os femoris should be flattish, and projected backward, to give advantage to the muscles that extend the tibia, by setting the center of motion backward: which mechanism, though it equally lessens the power of those muscles which bend this joint, is yet of great service, because the extending muscles move this joint under the weight

of

of the whole body, but the flexors only raiſe the legs; and as no head or ſocket moves ſo eaſily as round ones, here ſeems to be ſome proviſion made againſt the inconvenience of a flattiſh head and cavity, by having the friction made upon two ſurfaces, the os femoris upon the looſe cartilages, and the looſe cartilages upon the tibia. This contrivance is practiſed by mechanics, where the friction of the joints of any of their machines is great, as between the parts of hook-hinges of heavy gates, and between the male and female ſcrews of large vices, where they uſually place a looſe ring.

THERE are other cartilages which ſerve to give ſhape to parts. Of this ſort are the ciliary cartilages at the edges of the eye-lids, the cartilages of the outer ears, and thoſe which compoſe the lower part of the noſe, which have this particular advantage in theſe places, that they ſupport and ſhape the parts as well as bones do, and without being liable to be broke; and to theſe might be added thoſe of the larynx, but they do not belong properly to the ſceleton.

BONES that are articulated for motion are tied together by very ſtrong ligaments, to prevent their diſlocating, which alſo ſurround the joints to contain their lubricating mucus. The thickneſs and ſtrength of theſe ligaments are proportioned to the actions of the ſeveral joints, and their lengths are no more than ſufficient to allow a proper quantity of motion; but the forms of them

are

are different according to the different actions of the several joints.

The bones of the limbs that move to all ſides have ligaments like purſes, which ariſe from or near the edges of the ſockets of the receiving bones, and are inſerted all round the received bones a little below their heads. The beginnings of theſe ligaments, from the edges of the ſockets of the ſcapula and os innominatum, are very hard, almoſt cartilaginous, which ſerves in the ſcapula to make a larger ſocket, and ſuch an one as will alter its figure as the bone moves, for the reaſon I have mentioned in the looſe cartilage of the knee: for the head of the os humeri not being an exact portion of a ſphere, requires ſuch a ſocket, and the hard part of this ligament of the ſocket of the os innominatum makes the ſocket deeper than the ſemidiameter of the ſocket, by which means the articulation is made ſtronger without any hindrance to motion, becauſe it will give way to the neck of the os femoris when it preſſes againſt it; and the thigh bone being more diſpoſed to be diſlocated upwards than any other way, the upper ſide of this burſal ligament is made exceeding ſtrong to prevent ſuch an accident. From the lower edge of the acetabulum or ſocket of the os innominatum ariſes a ligament about an inch long, called teres, or rotundum, which length is neceſſary for that quantity of motion which this joint has in human bodies; it alſo hinders the os femoris from diſlocating upwards, but downwards

it

it will ſuffer it to go far out of the ſocket; but in brutes the head of the os femoris being oblong, and the cavity ſuitable, there can be only a rotatory motion, which in effect will be very little more than that kind of motion which is called bending and extending; and this never removing the end of the head of the bone far in the ſocket, a ſhort ligament is enough for it, and will better keep the bone in its place; and therefore it is that theirs is ſo ſhort. This ligament in men may alſo ſerve to preſs the gland in the bottom of the acetabulum or ſocket.

THE ligaments of thoſe joints which admit only of flexion and extenſion, differ from the former in this, that they are much ſhorter and ſtronger at the ſides of the joints, and thinner backward and forward. Beſides theſe ligaments, in the middle and back part of the joint of the knee, are two very ſtrong ligaments, which ariſe from a proceſs at the end of the tibia. They croſs each other in ſuch a manner, as is beſt to ſecure the joint from being diſplaced any way; they alſo hinder the extenſors of the tibia from pulling that bone too far forwards, and are ſo collected to the ſemilunar cartilages, as to move them as the joint moves; beſides theſe, in this joint is another ſmall one, which ariſes from the os femoris, and ends in the fatty membrane which it ſupports. The knee, I think, cannot be completely diſlocated without breaking the croſs ligaments: I have ſeen this caſe but once, the

the bone indeed was eaſily reſtored to its place, but to no purpoſe.

The bones of the carpus and tarſus are tied together by ligaments running promiſcuouſly upon their ſurfaces from one to another; which at the under ſide of the tarſus are vaſtly ſtrong, becauſe they ſupport the whole body; theſe ligaments together contain the mucus for all thoſe joints. There is alſo to the carpus a ſtrong ligament, which runs from the fifth bone to the eighth, and the proceſs of the fourth bone: the proper uſe of this is, to bind down the tendons of the muſcles that bend the fingers.

The proceſſus dentatus of the ſecond vertebra is tied to the ſcull by a ligament, and kept cloſe to the forepart of the firſt vertebra by another in that vertebra, that it may not bruiſe the ſpinal marrow; and when either this ligament or proceſs is broke, it makes that ſort of broken neck which is attended with ſudden death. All the bones of the vertebra, and every joint that is without motion, and not joined by a ſuture, as the oſſa innominata with each other, and the os ſacrum with the oſſa innominata, are joined by intervening ligaments, or, as they are commonly called, cartilages. The oſſa innominata are alſo tied by very ſtrong ligaments which run from the back parts of the ſpines of the oſſa ilia to the os ſacrum, and other ligaments which go from the os ſacrum and os coccygis to the acute and obtuſe proceſſes of the oſſa iſ-

chia:

chia: theſe ligaments ſerve alſo for origins of muſcles. Towards the great foramen of the oſſa innominata the acetabulum has a deep notch, from the one ſide to the other of which runs a ligament which completes the ſocket; this ligament is ſometimes oſſified: a ligament ſomewhat like this there is between the proceſſes of the ſcapula.

FROM the edge of the ilium to that of the os pubis, runs a ligament which is contiguous to, and appears to be a part of, the tendons of the muſcles of the abdomen; its uſe is to cover the iliac veſſels as they deſcend to the thigh. Under this ligament, together with the veſſels, I have often ſeen a rupture of matter, and, I think, ſometimes of the gut, from the abdomen into the anterior part of the thigh, immediately below the groin; however, I dare affirm this to be a poſſible caſe.

IT is generally agreed, that the ligaments are inſenſible; and the reaſon aſſigned is, that they would elſe be injured by ordinary motions. But they are much better contrived; ſeeing none of them, not even thoſe which lie between the vertebræ, are ſubject to attrition; but the other, experience ſhews, are capable of very acute pains; there being not any thing our patients more grievouſly complain of, than collections of matter within theſe parts, or ſharp medicines applied to them, when laid bare.

EVERY joint, where the bones are faced with a cartilage for a ſliding motion, is furniſhed with ſmall glands, which ſeparate a mucilaginous matter

ter for the lubricating of the ends of the bones, that they may move eaſily upon one another; and that there may be no waſte of this neceſſary fluid, it is contained in the inveſting ligaments; which, for this very reaſon, are no where divided, except to communicate with the ligaments of the tendons.

These glands are generally ſeated in a little fat near the inſertion of the ligaments, that they may be compreſſed by them when the joints are in motion; which is a proper time to have their fluid preſſed out. The moſt conſiderable parcel of theſe glands, with their fat, are ſeen in the joint of the knee, and the largeſt gland of this ſort is found in the ſinus at the bottom of the acetabulum of the os innominatum, and is compreſſed by the ligamentum teres.

The diſeaſes of the joints either happen from ulcers in the lubricating glands, which, pouring out matter that cannot be diſcharged, foul the ends of the bones, or elſe form ſwellings in the ends of the reſpective bones. Either of theſe in time create exceſſive pain, which appears to me to be chiefly in the ligaments of the joints, notwithſtanding what has been ſaid of the inſenſibility of theſe parts. When a joint is much ſwelled and painful, without external inflammation, it is vulgarly called a white ſwelling, and more properly ſo than ſpina ventoſa. It is ſometimes in the beginning cured by evacuations, but when the limb waſtes below the ſwelling, and the fingers or toes of the limb

grow

grow thinner at their joints, and loſe their ſhape, the caſe then is abſolutely irrecoverable. Sometimes the ends of the bones erode, then join together and form an anchyloſis, which, though a ſevere diſeaſe of itſelf, yet it is often a remedy of one that is much worſe. In like manner the bones of the hands and feet, when they are ulcerated, ſometimes unite, and are thus preſerved from total ruin. But there is one caſe of a white ſwelling that is amazing, where the pain is ſo great that we are forced to take off the limb, and yet neither find upon diſſection the ligaments or glands diſeaſed, nor matter in the joint, nor the bones carious, or any diſeaſed appearance, except that the ends of the bones are a little larger and ſofter.

TAB. I.

A, The ſceleton of a child twenty months old, in which all the bones differ in ſhape from thoſe of an adult. The ſcull is much larger in proportion, and the bones of the limbs without thoſe roughneſſes and unevenneſſes which afterwards appear; their texture is every where more looſe and ſpongy, and their outlines what the painters call tame and inſipid; their extremities are ſeparate and formed cartilaginous, which is accurately diſtinguiſhed in the plates by the manner of graving.

B, The thigh bone of a man, ſawed through, in the middle of which is ſeen the cavity which contains the oily marrow, and at the extremities the leſſer cells, which contain the bloody marrow. The white line acroſs the head of this bone, beginning at the fingers of the ſceleton, is the place where the epiphyſis and the bone are united. A like line, acroſs the lower end of this bone, ſhews there the ſame thing.

C, The os bregmatis of a fœtus ſix months old, which ſhews the fibres oſſifying from the centre to the circumference.

TAB. II.

TAB.I.

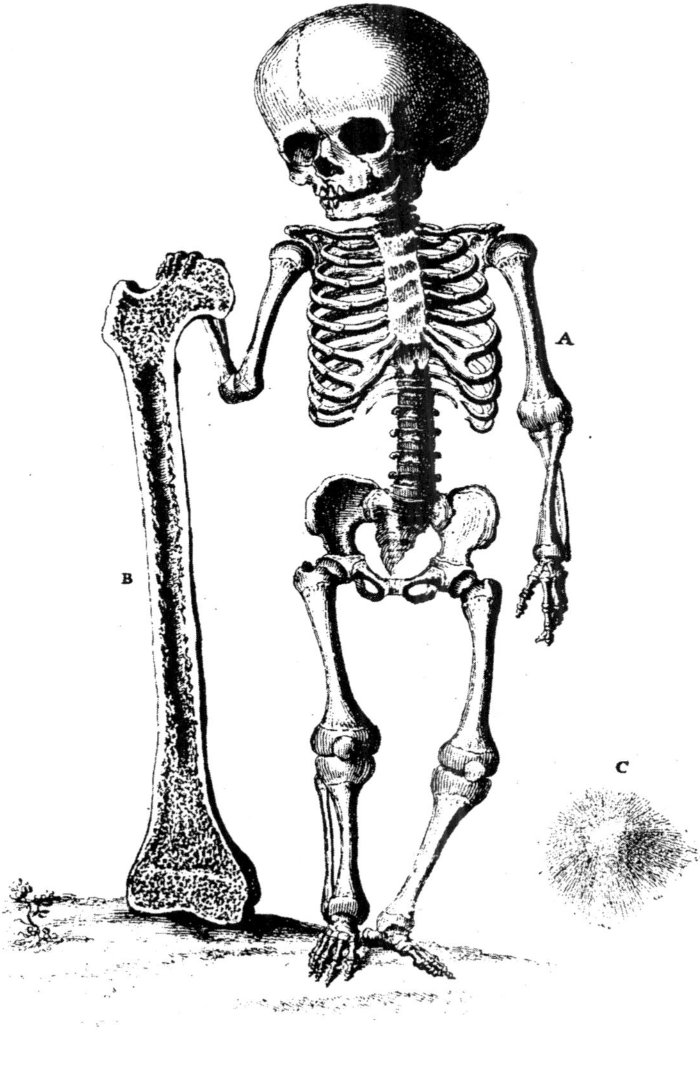

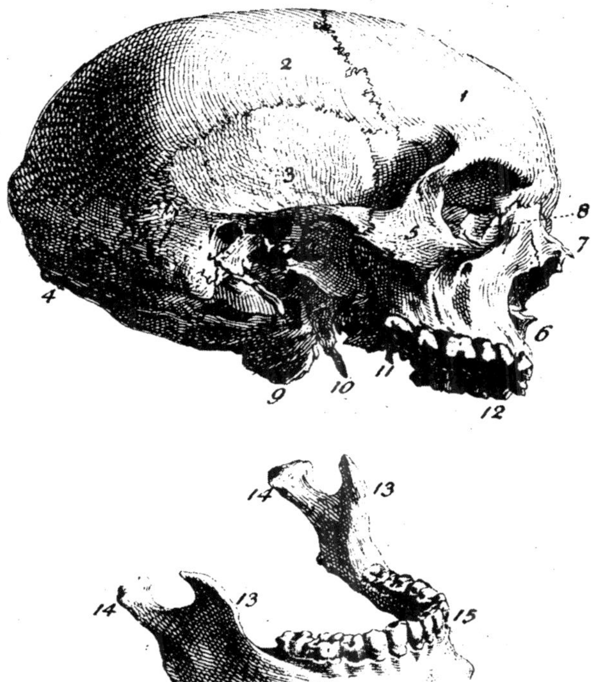
1
2
3
4
5
6
7
8
9
10
11
12
13
14
13
14
13
15

TAB II.

1 Os frontis.
2 Os bregmatis.
3 Os temporis.
4 Os occipitis.
5 Os malæ.
6 Os maxillæ ſuperioris.
7 Os naſi.
8 Os planum.
9 Proceſſus maſtoideus.
10 Proceſſus ſtyloides.
11 Proceſſus pterygoides.
12 Dentes.
13 Proceſſus coronalis.
14 Proceſſus condyloides.
15 Dentes.

TAB. III.

1 Os frontis.
2 Os bregmatis.
3 Os occipitis.
4 Sella turcica.
5 A process of the os sphenoides, making part of the septum nasi.
6 A process of the os ethmoides, making part of the septum nasi.
7 Vomer.
8 Crista galli, before which is seen in shadow the sinus frontalis.
9 The cornua of the os sphenoides.
10 Sella turcica.
11 Os frontis.
12 Crista galli and os ethmoides.
13 Sinus frontales.
14 Sella turcica.
15 The fifth foramen
16 Processus jugales.
17 Os petrosum.
18 Foramen magnum.
19 The outside of the os occipitis.

TAB. IV.

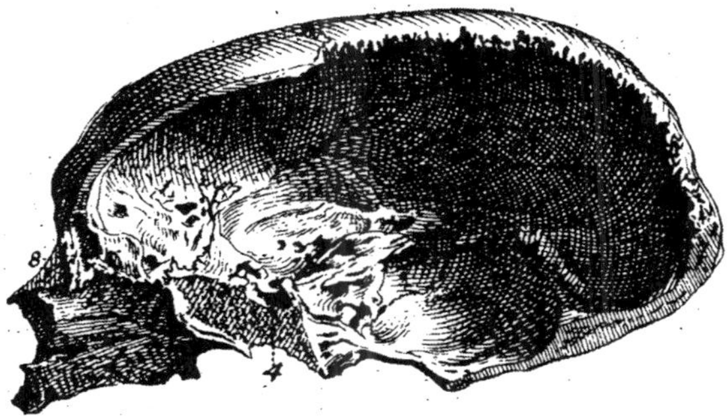
8
4

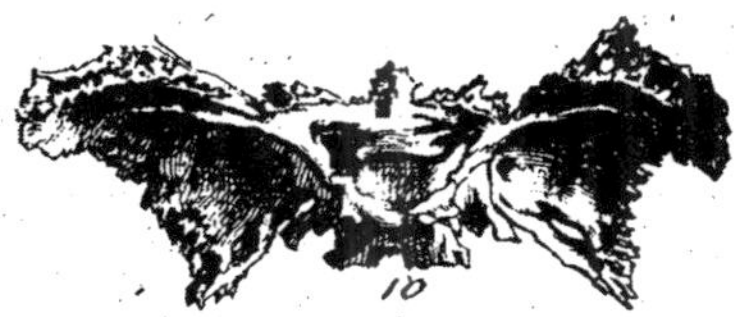
10

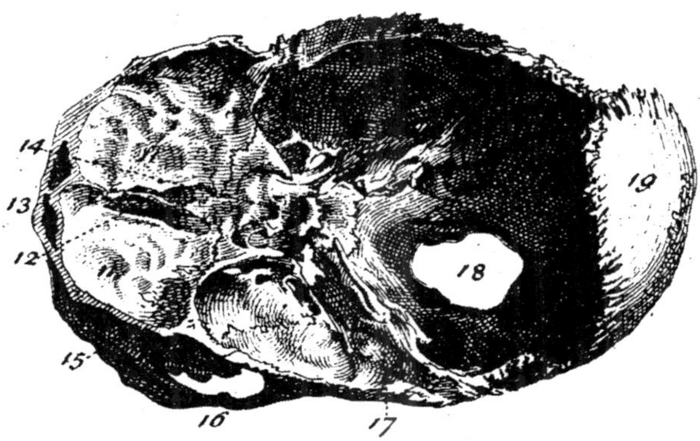
14
13
12
11
11
15
16
17
18
19

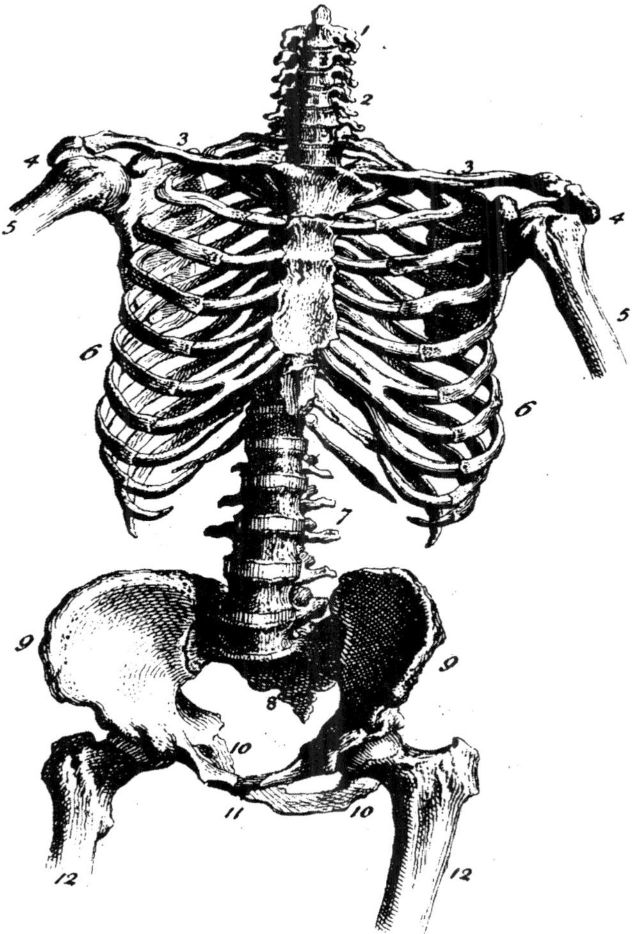
1
2
3
3
4
4
5
5
6
6
7
8
9
9
10
10
11
12
12

TAB. IV.

1 The ſecond vertebra of the neck.
2 The tranſverſe proceſſes of the vertebræ of the neck.
3 Clavicula.
4 The proceſſus acromion of the ſcapula.
5 Os humeri.
6 The ribs.
7 The tranſverſe proceſſes of the vertebræ of the loins.
8 The os ſacrum and os coccygis.
9 Os ileum.
10 Os iſchium.
11 Os pubis.
12 Os femoris.

TAB. V.

1 The under ſide of the firſt vertebra of the neck.
2 A ſide view of the ſecond vertebra.
3 The proceſſus dentatus of the ſecond vertebra.
4 The under ſide of the oblique proceſs.
5 The ſpinal proceſs,
6 The under ſide of the body of the ſeventh vertebra of the neck.
7 The tranſverſe proceſſes.
8 The oblique proceſſes.
9 The ſpinal proceſs.
10 The ſpinal proceſs of the ſecond vertebra of the back.
11 The under and fore ſide of the body of the vertebra.
12 The tranſverſe proceſſes.
13 The upper oblique proceſſes of the third vertebra of the back.
14 The tranſverſe proceſſes.
15 The ſpinal proceſs.
16 The body of the third vertebra of the loins.
17 The tranſverſe proceſſes.
18 The upper oblique proceſſes.
19 The ſpinal proceſs.

TAB.V.

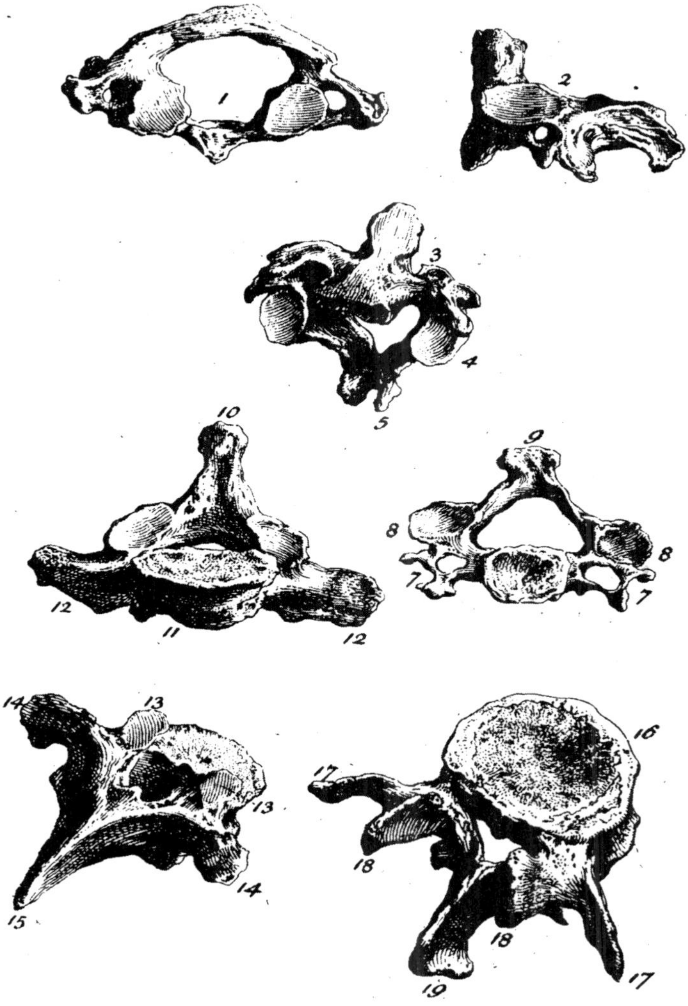

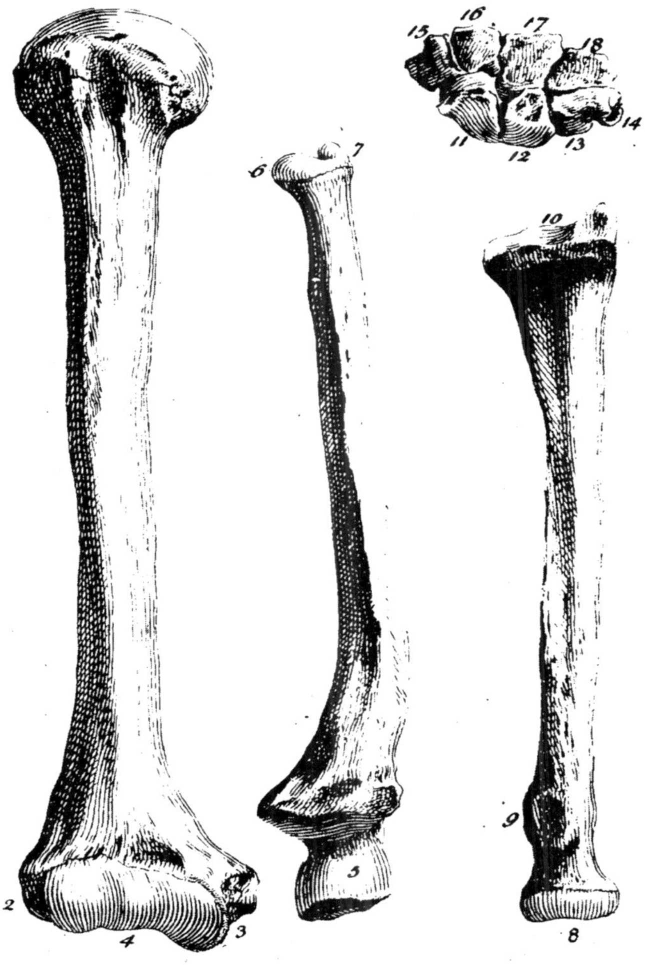
2
3
4
5
6
7
8
9
10
11
12
13
14
15
16
17
18

TAB. VI.

1 The head of the os humeri.
2 The outer extuberance.
3 The inner extuberance.
4 That part which joins with the ulna.
5 The olecranon of the ulna.
6 The lower end of the ulna which joins to the radius.
7 Processus styloides.
8. The upper of end of the radius.
9 The tubercle.
10 The part of the radius which joins with the carpus.
11, 12, 13, 14, 15, 16, 17, 18, The eight bones of the carpus.

TAB. VII.

1 Radius.
2 Ulna.
3 Carpus.
4 The three bones of the thumb.
5 The four bones of the metacarpus.
6 The three bones of the fingers.

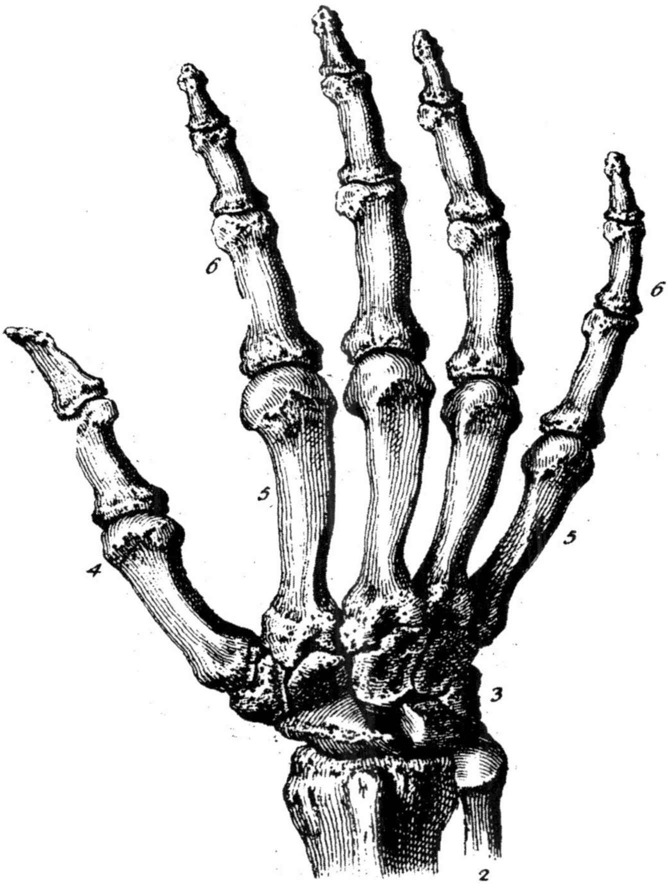
6
6
5
5
4
3
1
2

TAB.VIII.

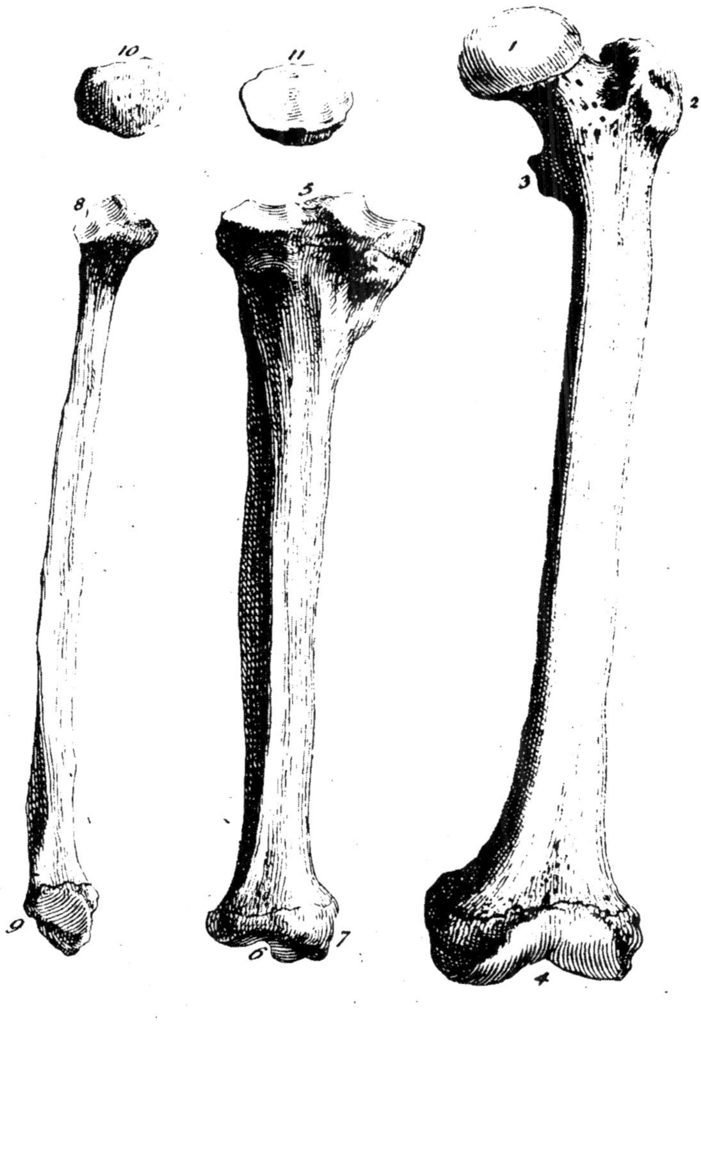

TAB. VIII.

1 The head of the os femoris.
2 The great trochanter.
3 The leſſer trochanter.
4 The lower end which articulates with the tibia.
5 The upper end of the tibia.
6 The lower end of the tibia.
7 The proceſs which makes the inner ankle.
8 The upper end of the fibula.
9 The lower end which makes the outer ankle.
10 The outſide of the patella.
11 The inſide of the patella.

TAB. IX.

1 Aſtragalus.
2 Os calcis.
3 Os naviculare.
4, 5, 6, Oſſa cuneiforma.
7 Os cuboides.
8 The five bones of the metatarſus.
9 The two bones of the great toe.
10 The three bones of the leſſer toes.

TAB. X.

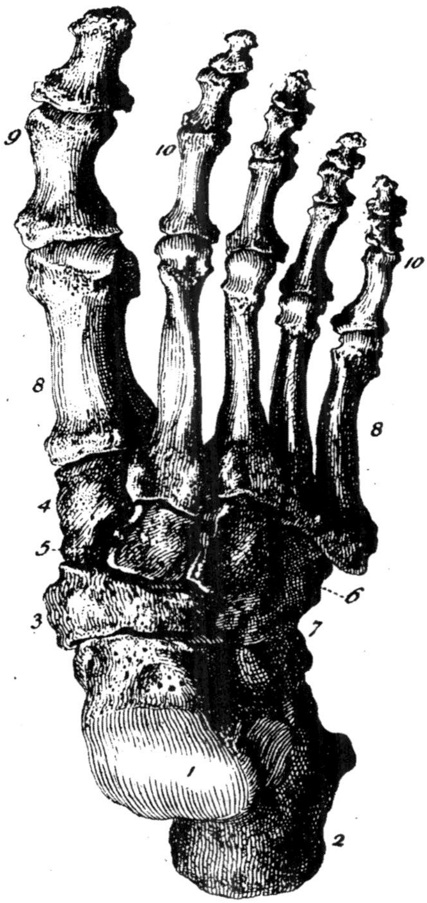
9
10
10
8
8
4
5
6
3
7
1
2

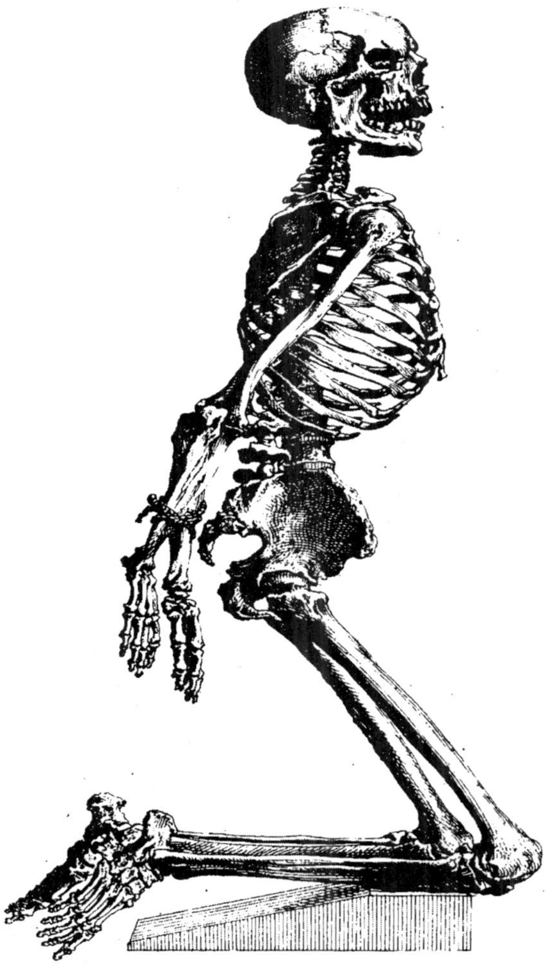

TAB. X.

A ſceleton of an adult put into this poſture to ſhew it in a greater ſcale. It was thought better not to figure it, all theſe bones being explained in former plates, and the deſign of this being to ſhew them together, without being defaced with references.

THE

THE ANATOMY OF THE Human Body.

BOOK II.

CHAPTER I.

Introduction to the muſcles.

THE muſcles are moving powers, applied to perform the ſeveral motions of the body; which they do by contracting their length, and thereby bringing the parts to which they are fixed nearer together. The immoveable or leaſt moved part any muſcle is fixed to, is uſually called its origin, and the other its inſertion; but muſcles that have their two ends equally liable to be moved, may have either called their origins or inſertions.

EACH

EACH muſcle is made up of a number of ſmall fibres, which BORELLI and others have thought to be ſtrings of bladders, and have endeavoured to account for muſcular motion by an expanſion made from an influx of blood and animal ſpirits into theſe bladders; but as the muſcles do not increaſe their bulk ſenſibly in contracting, there needs no more to be ſaid to refute this hypotheſis. But another great author thought that in this way the muſcles might be contracted by a ſwelling, ſcarce ſenſible, if the bladders were but very ſmall: For, ſays he, ſuppoſing a bladder of any determined bigneſs can raiſe a weight a foot, a hundred bladders, whoſe diameters are each a hundredth part of the former, will raiſe the weight to the ſame height. But the force of inflation and the ſwelling of all together will be ten thouſand times leſs, and it will alſo raiſe ten thouſand times leſs weight, which he has not obſerved; therefore not one ſuch ſtring of bladders, but ten thouſand, muſt be applied to do the ſame thing that the one bladder will do; and they will have the ſame ſwelling; otherwiſe it would be eaſy to ſhew how to make a perpetuum mobile of almoſt any force.

THE muſcles are of two ſorts, viz. rectilineal, and penniform. The former have their fibres almoſt parallel, in the ſame or near the ſame direction with the axis of the muſcle; and the latter have their fibres joined, in an oblique direction, to a tendon paſſing in or near the axis, or on their outſide.

THE

The rectilineal muscles, if their origins and insertions are in little compass, are never of any considerable thickness, unless they are very long, because the outward fibres would compress the inner ones, and make them almost useless; and therefore every rectilineal muscle, whose inner fibres are compressed by the outer, have their inner fibres longer than the external, that they may be capable of equal quantity of contraction.

The penniform muscles, though they are in a manner free from the inconvenience of one fibre compressing another, and though by the obliquity of their fibres, nothing is abated of their moment, (for in all cases, just so much more weight as rectilineal fibres will raise than oblique ones, the oblique will move their weight with so much greater velocity than the rectilineal; which is making their moments equal: so that in the structure of an animal, like all mechanic engines, whatever is gained in strength is lost in velocity, and whatever is gained in velocity is lost in strength) yet the fibres of the penniform muscles becoming more and more oblique as they contract, their strength decreases, and their velocity increases, which makes them less uniform in their actions than the rectilineal muscles; wherefore it seems that nature never uses a penniform muscle where a rectilineal muscle can be used; and the cases in which a rectilineal muscle cannot be used, are where the shape of a muscle is such as that the inward fibres would be too much compreſſed, or where rectilineal fibres could not have a lever to act with, ſuitable to their quantity of contraction, which is the caſe of all the long muſcles of the fingers and toes. For every muſcle muſt be inſerted or paſs over the centre of motion of the joint it moves, at a diſtance ſuitable to its quantity of contraction, and the quantity of motion in the joint moved; for if it was inſerted too near, then the motion of the joint would be performed before the muſcle is contracted all that it can; if too far off, the muſcle will have done contracting before the whole motion of the joint is made. And though the quickneſs and quantity of motion in a muſcle will be, cæteris paribus, as the length of its fibres; (for if a fibre four inches long will contract one inch in a given time, a fibre eight inches long will contract two inches in the ſame time; and the ſtrength of a muſcle or power to raiſe a weight, cæteris paribus, will be as the number of its fibres; for if one fibre will raiſe a grain weight, twenty fibres will raiſe twenty grains:) nevertheleſs, two muſcles of equal magnitude, one long, and the other ſhort, will both move the ſame weight with the ſame velocity when applied to a bone; becauſe the levers they act with muſt be as their lengths, and therefore the penniform and ſhort thick muſcles are never applied to a bone for the ſake of ſtrength, nor long fibred muſcles for quickneſs; for whatever is gained by the form of the muſcle, whether ſtrength

or

or quicknefs, muft be loft by their infertions into the bone, or elfe the mufcles muft not act all they can, or the bones have lefs motion than they are made for.

In the limbs feveral mufcles pafs over two joints, both of which are liable to move at once, with force proportionable to the levers they act with upon each joint; but either joint being fixed by an antagonift mufcle, the whole force of fuch mufcles will be exerted upon the other joint; which in that cafe may be moved with a velocity equal to what is in both joints, when thefe mufcles act upon both at once. This mechanifm is of great ufe in the limbs, as I fhall fhew in the proper places.

That only we call the proper ufe and action of any mufcle which it has without the neceffary affiftance of any other mufcle, and what that is in a mufcle moving a joint we may always know in any fituation, and with what force it acts, cæteris paribus, by dropping a line, from the centre of motion of the joint it moves, perpendicular into the axis of the mufcle; but in a joint which admits only of flexion and extenfion, this line muft alfo be perpendicular to the axis of motion in that joint, and the action of the mufcles will be in the direction of that perpendicular line, and the force with which it acts in any fituation will be, cæteris paribus, as the length of that perpendicular line.

 Each

Each muſcle, ſo far as it is diſtinct, and is moved againſt any part, is covered with a ſmooth membrane to make the friction eaſy; but where they are externally tendinous, thoſe tendons are often ſmooth enough to make ſuch a covering needleſs. Beſides this membrane there is another, known by the name of faſcia tendinoſa, which deſerves to be particularly conſidered. The ſtrong one on the outſide of the thigh, which belongs to the faſcialis and gluteus muſcles, is of great uſe in raiſing the gluteus farther from the centre of motion of the joint it moves, to increaſe its force: in like manner the faſcia detached from the tendon of the biceps cubiti alters its direction for the ſame purpoſe, but thoſe on the outſide of the tibia and cubit, &c. are only flat tendons from which the fibres of the muſcles ariſe as from the bones. There are alſo in many places ſuch tendons between the muſcles, from which each muſcle ariſes in like manner; for the bones themſelves are not ſufficient to give origin to half the fibres of the muſcles that belong to them; beſides, if all the fibres had riſe from the bones, they muſt have been liable to compreſs one another very inconveniently.

CHAPTER

CHAPTER II.

Of the muscles.

OBLIQUUS DESCENDENS arises fleshy from near the extremities of the eight inferior ribs, the upper part of its origin being indented with the serratus major anticus, and the lower lying under a small portion of the latissimus dorsi. It is inserted fleshy into the upper part of the spine of the ilium, and by a broad flat tendon (which firmly adheres to a like tendon of the following muscle as they pass over the rectus) into the os pubis, and linea alba, which is a strong tendinous line extended from the os pubis to the sternum, between the musculi recti.

OBLIQUUS ASCENDENS arises fleshy under the former muscle from the spine of the ilium, and is inserted fleshy in the cartilages of the three lowest ribs, and by a flat tendon into the sternum, and linea alba, together with the tendon of the foregoing muscle. The line in which these two tendons join on the outside of the rectus muscle, is called semilunaris: and though so much of this muscle as is inserted fleshy runs obliquely upward, yet the middle and lower part is directed transverse and downward; and beside the tendon, which it unites with the obliquus descendens, it often detaches another near the sternum to be inserted with the transversalis under the rectus.

Pyramidalis arifes from the os pubis, and is inferted into the linea alba, about three or four inches below the navel: this and its fellow are often wanting.

Rectus arifes tendinous from the os pubis, but flefhy when the pyramidales are wanting, and is inferted into the lower part of the fternum, near the cartilago enfiformis. This mufcle is divided into four or five portions by tranfverfe tendinous interfections, that it might conveniently bend when the body is bowed forwards, though this mufcle fhould be then in action; and thefe interfections are chiefly above the navel, where it is moft liable to be bent: befides, being thus divided, its chief preffure will not be in its middle, but under the feveral bellies of the mufcle, and the greateft below the navel, where is the longeft flefhy belly of this mufcle, and where the parts in the abdomen feem to want moft to be fupported.

Transversalis arifes by a flat tendon from the tranfverfe proceffes of the lumbal vertebræ, and flefhy from the infide of the ribs below the diaphragm, and from the fpine of the ilium; then, becoming a flat tendon, it paffes under the rectus to its infertion into the linea alba. Between this tendon and the peritoneum fometimes water is found in great quantities, which diftemper is called the dropfy in the duplicature of the peritoneum; which fhews this membrane has been miftaken for part of the peritoneum.

These

These five pair of muſcles all conſpire to compreſs the parts contained in the abdomen. The obliquus deſcendens on the right ſide, and aſcendens on the left acting together, turn the upper part of the trunk of the body towards the left, and vice verſa; but the trunk is chiefly turned upon the thighs; the recti bend the body forward, and pull the ſternum downward in expiration; the two oblique muſcles and the tranſverſe on each ſide near the groins, are perforated to let through the proceſſus vaginalis with the ſpermatic veſſels. Theſe perforations are diſtant from each other, ſo as to ſuffer the veſſels to deſcend conveniently into the ſcrotum: this way the inteſtines or the omentum deſcend in ruptures.

Cremaster testis is a ſmall portion of fibres which ariſes from the ilium, and appears to be part of the obliqnus aſcendens muſcle, 'till it meets with the ſpermatic veſſels at their coming out of the abdomen, where it begins to deſcend with them by the ſide of the proceſſus vaginalis, to the teſticle, over which it is looſely expanded. This muſcle is too ſmall to be plainly diſcovered in emaciated bodies.

Erector penis ariſes from the os iſchium, and is inſerted into the crus penis near the os pubis. It is ſaid, by preſſing the penis againſt the os pubis to compreſs the vena ipſius penis, and hinder the reflux of blood, whereby the penis becomes extended ed and erect; but it does not appear to me to be well contrived for that use.

Accelerator urinæ. This, with its fellow, are but one muscle. It arises tendinous from the ossa ischia, and fleshy from the sphincter ani; or, according to Mr. Cowper, from the superior part of the urethra as it passes under the os pubis: and thence, being expanded over the bulb of the urethra, it afterwards divides, and is inserted into the penis. The use of this muscle is not to accelerate the urine, for that is propell'd by the detrusor urinæ, or muscular coat of the bladder, but to protrude the semen, which is done only by this; and it being seated opposite to the os pubis, it seems to be much better fitted to be a relaxer of the penis, by pulling it from the os pubis, than the erector is for the office assigned it.

Transversalis penis is that part of the former muscle which arises from the ossa ischia.

Sphincter vesicæ urinariæ is a small portion of muscular fibres, not easily to be distinguished, running round the neck of the bladder to prevent the involuntary effusion of urine.

Detrusor urinæ is the muscular coat of the bladder; its fibres are differently disposed; but chiefly terminating in the sphincter vesicæ, whereby it not only presses the urine forward, but, when the bladder is full, becomes an antagonist to the sphincter, acting almost at right angles.

Ere-

ERECTOR CLITORIDIS ariſes from the iſchium, and is inſerted into the crus clitoridis, like the erector penis in men, and is ſaid to cauſe erection in the ſame manner.

SPHINCTER VAGINÆ is an order of muſcular fibres, intermixed with membranous fibres, ſurrounding the vagina uteri near its orifice; it is connected to the oſſa pubis and ſphincter ani; its uſe is to conſtringe the orifice of the vagina, to preſs out a liquor from the glands of the vagina, and embrace the penis in coition.

DR. DOUGLAS mentions two pair of muſcles of the vagina, of his own diſcovering, which I have never diſſected, and will therefore give them in his own words; "The firſt ariſes from the inner edge "of the os pubis mid-way between the iſchion and "the beginning of the crus clitoridis, is inſerted "into the vagina; the ſecond ariſes tendinous and "fleſhy from the os pubis internally in common "with the levator ani, is inſerted into the upper "part of the vagina at the ſide of the meatus uri- "narius or collum veſicæ."

SPHINCTER ANI is a muſcle near two inches in breadth, ſurrounding the anus to cloſe it, and to prevent involuntary falling out of the fæces.

LEVATOR ANI, by Dr. DOUGLAS called two pair of muſcles, but Mr. COWPER deſcribes the whole as one muſcle only, which ariſes from the oſſa iſchii, pubis, and ſacrum within the pelvis, and is inſerted round the lower end of the rectum inteſtinum.

FISTULÆ in ano, that are within this muſcle, generally run in the direction of the gut, and may be laid open into the gut with great ſafety; but thoſe fiſtulæ, or rather abſceſſes, that are frequently formed on the outſide of the ſphincter, and uſually ſurround it, all but where this muſcle is connected to the penis, cannot be opened far into the gut, without totally dividing the ſphincter, which authors ſay, renders the ſphincter ever after incapable of retaining the excrement. One inſtance of this kind I have known; but Mr. BERBECK of York, an excellent ſurgeon, and particularly famous for this operation, has aſſured me, that he has often been forced to divide the ſphincter, which has made the patients unable to hold their excrements during their cure, but the wounds being healed, they have retained them as well as ever.

COCCYGEI ariſe from the acute proceſſes of the oſſa iſchii, and are inſerted into the os coccygis, which they pull forward.

OCCIPITO-FRONTALIS, is a muſcle with four fleſhy bellies, commonly named frontales and occipitales. It ariſes behind each ear from the os occipitis, and ſoon becoming tendinous, paſſes under the hairy ſcalp to the forehead, where it becomes broad and fleſhy, adhering to the ſkin, and is inſerted into the upper part of the orbicular muſcles of the eyelids into the os frontis near the noſe, and by two proceſſes into the bones of the noſe. When this muſcle acts from the back part, it pulls the

ſkin

ſkin of the forehead upward, and wrinkles it tranſverſe, and in ſome perſons the hairy ſcalp backwards; but when the forepart of it acts, it draws the ſkin with the eyebrows downward, and towards the noſe when we frown. The tendon of this muſcle has been miſtaken for a membrane, and been called pericranium, and the true pericranium, perioſteum.

ELEVATOR AURICULÆ ariſes from the tendon of the occipito-frontalis, and is inſerted into the upper part of the ear that is connected to the head.

RETRACTOR AURICULÆ ariſes by one, two, or three ſmall portions from the temporal bone above the mammillary proceſs, and is inſerted into the ear to pull it backward.

ORBICULARIS PALPEBRARUM ſurrounds the eyelids on the edge of the orbit, and is fixed to the ſutura tranſverſalis at the great corner of the eye; it ſhuts the eyelids, eſpecially in winking. That part of this muſcle that lies under the eyebrow is very much intermixed with the occipito-frontalis; and under it, from the os frontis near the noſe, ariſes a ſmall portion of diſtinct fibres which end in this muſcle, and, I think, are a part of it; nevertheleſs, from the effect of their action, are not improperly called muſculus corrugator.

CILIARIS is a very ſmall portion of this muſcle, next the ciliary cartilages of the eyelids.

ELE-

Elevator palpebræ superioris rectus riſes above the optic nerve, from the perioſteum at the bottom of the orbit, as do alſo the five following muſcles, and is inſerted into the whole ciliary cartilage of the upper eyelid by a very thin flat tendon.

Elevator oculi ariſes from the bottom of the orbit, between the optic nerve and the foregoing muſcle, and is inſerted in the upper part of the tunica ſclerotis of the eye, near the cornea.

Depressor oculi ariſes, and is inſerted directly oppoſite to the laſt deſcribed muſcle.

Adductor oculi ariſes from the bottom of the orbit, near the optic nerve internally, and is inſerted into the tunica ſclerotis on the ſide next the noſe.

Abductor oculi has both its origin and inſertion directly oppoſite to the adductor.

Obliquus superior ſeu trochlearis ariſes between the elevator and adductor oculi at the bottom of the orbit, thence aſcending by the ſutura tranſverſalis, becomes a round tendon, which paſſing through a pulley at the upper and inner part of the orbit near its edge, is inſerted near the bottom of the globe of the eye, which it pulls upward and inward, and thereby directs the pupil outward and downward.

Obliquus inferior ariſes from the os maxillæ ſuperioris, at the edge of the orbit; thence paſſing over the depreſſor is inſerted near the abductor

ductor at the bottom of the eye, but not ſo low as the inſertion of the obliquus ſuperior: it turns the pupil upward and outward.

THESE muſcles are inſerted with great advantage to move a ſmall weight, and are very long, that the eye may be moved with ſufficient quickneſs. The two oblique muſcles are an axis to the motions of the other four, and acting ſtrongly againſt them, which action I take to be what is vulgarly called ſtraining the eye, may, I think, bring the cryſtalline humour nearer to the retina, and poſſibly may make the cryſtalline humour more flat to fit the eye for objects at a great diſtance. For this end it ſeems to me that there are ſix muſcles thus diſpoſed, when three might be ſufficient to turn the eye every way, if it was in a proper fixed ſocket; and it ſeems alſo, that while the muſcles are all thus in action, the ſuperior oblique in each eye ſets the pupil farther from the noſe, while the inferior oblique directs it upward; the firſt of which actions is always neceſſary, and the latter often ſo, when we look with both eyes at very diſtant objects; and when the two oblique muſcles grow weak by age or diſeaſe, or ceaſe to act at all, as in paralytic caſes, and death, then the eye ſinks in the orbit.

SPHINCTER, OF CONSTRICTOR ORIS, ſurrounds the mouth about three fourths of an inch broad. This muſcle is very much intermixed with all the muſcles that are inſerted into it.

ELE-

Elevator labii superioris proprius ariſes from the bone of the upper jaw under the anterior and inferior part of the orbicularis palpebrarum, and uſually takes another ſmall beginning from the os malæ, which ſeems as if it was ſent off from the orbicularis palpebrarum; and paſſing down by the ſide of the noſe, into which it ſends ſome fibres, is inſerted into the upper part of the ſphincter oris. This raiſes the upper lip, and helps to dilate the noſtrils.

Depressor labii superioris proprius is a ſmall muſcle ariſing from the upper jaw, near the dentes inciſorii, and is inſerted into the upper part of the lip and root of the cartilages of the noſe; hence it is alſo a depreſſor of the noſe, which action conſtricts the noſtrils.

Depressor labii inferioris proprius ariſes broad from the lower jaw at the chin, and is ſoon inſerted into the ſphincter oris; the order of fibres in this ſeems not ſo conſpicuous as in the other muſcles of the face.

Elevator labii inferioris proprius ariſes from the lower jaw, near the dentes inciſorii, and is inſerted into the lower part of the lip.

Elevator labiorum communis ariſes from a depreſſed part of the ſuperior maxilla under the middle of the orbit, and is inſerted into the ſphincter muſcle near the corner of the mouth.

Depressor communis labiorum ariſes laterally from the lower jaw near the chin, and is inſerted

inſerted into the ſphincter oppoſite to the former.

Zygomaticus ariſes from the anterior part of the os zygoma or malæ, and frequently derives a portion of fibres from the orbicularis palpebrarum, thence running obliquely downwards. It is inſerted into the ſphincter at the corner of the mouth, betwixt the elevator communis and buccinator; it draws the corner of the mouth outward and upward. When this muſcle grows weak, the corner of the mouth ſinks, as may be obſerved in old perſons.

Buccinator ariſes from the proceſſus coronæ of the lower jaw, and paſſing contiguous to both jaws, is inſerted into the ſphincter muſcle at the corner of the mouth. It ſerves either to force breath out of the mouth, or thruſt the aliment between the teeth in maſtication, or to pull the corner of the mouth outward.

Platysma myoides ariſes looſely from over the pectoral and part of the deltoid muſcle, and running obliquely forward, is inſerted into the chin, and depreſſor muſcles of the lips. This muſcle being exceeding thin, a mere membrana carnoſa, ſerves to cover the unequal ſurface of the ſubjacent muſcles, and render the neck even; it alſo pulls down the corner of the mouth, and, from its inſertion at the chin, may contribute to the pulling down of the lower jaw.

Retractor alæ nasi is a very ſmall muſcle ariſing from the bone of the noſe, and is inſert-

 ed

ed into the ſkin and cartilage at the ſide of the noſe.

Mylohyoideus with its fellow, may be eſteemed one penniform or elſe a digaſtric muſcle. It ariſes from the linea aſpera on the inſide of the lower jaw and proceſſus innominatus, both ſides meeting at about right angles in a middle line upon the following muſcles. It is inſerted by a ſmall portion of fibres into the baſis of the os hyoides; it moves the tongue upward and forward, and alſo compreſſes the following muſcles, whereby they raiſe the tongue more commodiouſly, and alſo hinders them from drawing the baſis of the os hyoides into a right line betwixt the chin and ſternum at ſuch times as the ſtylohyoidei cannot act.

Geniohyoideus ariſes from the proceſſus innominatus of the lower jaw, under the foregoing muſcle, and is inſerted into the baſis of the os hyoides, which it pulls upward and forward. This, with its fellow, are for the moſt part but one muſcle.

Stylohyoideus ariſes from the proceſſus ſtyliformis, near its root, and paſſing contiguous to the horn of the os hyoides becomes inſerted laterally into its baſis. This muſcle is ſometimes perforated about the middle, by the tendon of the digaſtric muſcle of the lower jaw. Its uſe is to pull the os hyoides up and backward.

Coracohyoideus ariſes from the upper coſta of the ſcapula, near the proceſſus coracoides, and paſſing

paſſing under the maſtoideus muſcle becomes in that place a round tendon ; thence paſſing almoſt parallel to the following muſcle, is inſerted together with it into the baſis of the os hyoides ; this draws the os hyoides downward, and a little backward. I have once ſeen one of theſe muſcles wanting, and the ſternohyoideus ariſing from the middle of the clavicle on that ſide.

STENROHYOIDEUS ariſes from a roughneſs at the under part of the clavicula near the ſternum, and the cartilaginous part of the firſt rib ; and is inſerted into the baſis of the os hyoides, to pull it downward.

GENIOGLOSSUS ariſes from the proceſſus innominatus of the lower jaw, and is inſerted broad into the under part of the tongue, to pull it up and forward, and ſometimes has a ſmall inſertion into the os hyoides.

BASIOGLOSSUS ſeems a portion of the former muſcle ; it ariſes from the baſis of the os hyoides, and is inſerted into the tongue nearer its tip.

CERATOGLOSSUS ariſes from the horn of the os hyoides, and is inſerted laterally into the tongue near its root, to pull it downward and forward.

STYLOGLOSSUS ariſes from the extremity of the proceſſus ſtyliformis, and is inſerted into the tongue near the former to pull it up and backward. I have very often found another ſtyloid muſcle ſo inſerted, that I cannot tell whether to call it a muſcle of the tongue or pharynx.

THE

THE TONGUE is a muſcle made of fibres, longitudinal, circular, and tranſverſe, ſo intermixed as beſt to ſerve its ſeveral motions.

HYOTHYROIDEUS, or CERATOTHYROIDEUS, ariſes from part of the baſis, and the horn of the os hyoides, and is inſerted into the lower part of the cartilago thyroides, to pull it upward.

STERNOTHYROIDEUS ariſes from the inſide of the ſternum, and is inſerted with the former; it pulls the thyroid cartilage directly downward.

CRICOTHYROIDEUS ariſes from the anterior part of the cartilago cricoides, and running obliquely upward and outward, is ſoon inſerted into the inſide of the cartilago thyroides, which it pulls towards the cartilago cricoides. Both this muſcle and its fellow for the moſt part appear double.

CRICOARYTÆNOIDEUS POSTICUS ariſes from the back part of the cartilago cricoides, and is inſerted into the arytænoides to pull it backward.

CRICOARYTÆNOIDEUS LATERALIS ariſes laterally from the cartilago cricoides, and is inſerted laterally into the arytænoides. This, with its fellow, pull down each cartilage toward their origin, and thereby dilate the rimula.

THYROARYTÆNOIDEUS ariſes from the ſuperior, middle, and inner part of the cartilago thyroides, and is inſerted with the former into the arytænoides cartilage to dilate the rimula. Theſe two laſt deſcribed muſcles are not naturally divided, and therefore ought to be accounted but one muſcle.

ARY-

ARYTÆNOIDEUS is one ſingle muſcle, which ariſes from one arytænoidal cartilage, and is inſerted into the other, to draw them together, and cloſe the rimula. Theſe few ſmall muſcles of the tongue and larynx, with only one pipe, make a greater variety of notes and ſounds than can be made by artificial inſtruments, and that in a manner ſo little underſtood by us, and by organs ſo little differing from thoſe in quadrupeds, that, for aught we know of them, brutes might be as capable of all theſe ſounds as men.

STYLOPHARYNGÆUS ariſes from near the bottom of the proceſſus ſtyloides of the os petroſum, and running obliquely downward, is inſerted into the pharynx. This muſcle, with its fellow, pulls up and dilates the pharynx to receive the aliment.

OESOPAAGEUS ariſes like a wing from ſeveral parts of the ſcull, tongue, os hyoides, the cricoid and thyroid cartilages, and is inſerted into the pharynx. This, with its fellow, conſtringe the pharynx, and preſs the aliment down the gullet.

MUSCULUS VAGINALIS GULÆ is the muſcular coat of the gula.

PTERYGOPHARYNGÆUS is not a diſtinct muſcle, but the beginning of the pharynx near the proceſſus pterygoides of the ſphenoidal bone.

PTERYGOSTAPHYLINUS INTERNUS ariſes from the os ſphenoides, near the iter ad palatum, or euſtachian tube, and is inſerted into the uvula,

 which

which it pulls up while we breathe through the mouth, or ſwallow.

Pterygo-staphylinus externus ariſes by the ſide of the laſt deſcribed muſcle, and is alſo inſerted near it; but becomes its antogoniſt by being reflected on a pulley, over a proceſs at the lower part of the pterygoidal proceſſes of the ſphenoidal bone.

Glosso-staphylinus is a very ſmall portion of muſcular fibres, which paſs from the tongue to the palate, which it pulls down when we breathe through the noſe.

The palate itſelf is a ſort of double muſcle, whoſe action ſeems only to ſupport itſelf, and aſſiſt thoſe muſcles which pull it upwards.

Digastricus ariſes from the ſinus of the mamillary proceſs of the os temporis, and from a fleſhy belly, becoming a round tendon, paſſes through, and ſometimes under the ſtylohyoideus muſcle; and then, being tied down by a ligament to the os hyoides, grows fleſhy, and is ſo inſerted into the anterior part of the lower jaw internally. This muſcle's direction being altered by its being tied to the os hyoides, where it makes an angle, and not at its paſſage through the ſtylohyoideus, pulls the lower jaw downward with much greater force than otherwiſe it could have done; and being connected to the os hyoides, when it acts, it prevents the action of ſeveral muſcles which are concerned in ſwallowing, whence it is that we cannot ſwal-

low

low at the ſame time that we open the jaw, as thoſe brutes can whoſe digaſtric muſcles are not connected to that bone.

Temporalis ariſes from the os frontis, parietale, ſphenoides, malæ, and temporis, and, paſſing under the two proceſſes named os jugale, is inſerted externally into the proceſſus coronalis of the lower jaw, which it pulls upward. This muſcle is covered with a ſtrong tendinous faſcia.

Masseter ariſes from the lower edge of the os malæ or zygoma, and the proceſs which joins this from the temporal bone, and is inſerted into the outer part of the angle of the lower jaw, which it pulls up and forward. Theſe two laſt deſcribed muſcles having different directions, when they act together, make a ſteddy motion in the diagonal of their directions.

Pterygoideus internus ariſes from the proceſſus pterygoideus externus, and from the ſinus between the pterygoid proceſſes, and is inſerted internally into the angle of the lower jaw, which it pulls upward.

Pterygoideus externus ariſes from the os maxillare and os ſphenoides, near the root of the external pterygoid proceſs, and is inſerted internally into the proceſſus condyloides of the lower jaw, which it pulls to one ſide, and forwards, or acting with its fellow pulls the jaw directly forward.

Subclavius ariſes from the ſuperior part of the firſt rib, and is inſerted into more than half the underside of the clavicula next the scapula. Its use is to draw the clavicula toward the sternum, that they may not be severed in the motions of the scapula.

TRAPEZIUS arises from the os occipitis, and from a linea alba colli, from the spinal process of the last vertebra of the neck, and the ten uppermost of the back, and from a linea alba between all these processes; and is inserted into one third of the clavicle next the scapula, almost all the back part of the spine of the scapula, and as much of the processus acromion as lies between the spine of the scapula and the clavicle. This muscle draws the scapula directly backward.

IT is generally said by authors, that the several parts of this muscle act at different times, and so pull the scapula different ways, as obliquely upward, downward, or backward; but, I think, if that happened, it must necessarily divide this muscle into distinct portions, those that contract always separating from those that do not.

RHOMBOIDES arises tendinous under the former from the spinal process of the inferior vertebra of the neck, part of the linea alba colli, and from the spinal processes of the four or five uppermost vertebræ of the thorax, and is inserted into the basis of the scapula, which it pulls up and backward. The upper part of this muscle arising from the neck, is, in many bodies, by the motions of the neck, separated and made a distinct muscle.

ELE-

Elevator scapulæ arifes from the tranf-verfe proceffes of the four fuperior vertebræ of the neck, and is inferted into the upper angle of the fcapula.

Serratus minor anticus arifes under the pectoralis, from the third, fourth, and fifth ribs, and is inferted into the proceffus coracoides fcapulæ, which it pulls forward and downward. This mufcle is always faid to be an elevator of the ribs, though it arifes from the fcapula, which is fupported by the ribs.

Serratus major anticus arifes from the anterior part of the eight fuperior ribs, and is inferted into the bafis of the fcapula, which it draws forward, and by that means moves the focket of the fcapula upward. This mufcle has been always accounted an elevator coftarum, though each portion of it is nearly parallel to the rib it rifes from.

All the mufcles inferted into the bafis of the fcapula are alfo inferted into one another.

Pectoralis arifes from near two thirds of the clavicula, next the fternum, and all the length of the os pectoris, and from the cartilages of the ribs, and is inferted into the os humeri, between the biceps and the infertion of the deltoides. The ufe of it is to draw the arm forward. A fmall portion of the lower part of this mufcle is often confounded with the obliquus defcendens abdominis; and in fome bodies, neither the upper part, nor its tendon, can be eafily feparated from the deltoides; and in

 others,

others, even that part of it that arises from the clavicula is a distinct portion. Near the insertion of this muscle the fibres cross those from below, ending above in the arm, and those from above below, that the tendon of this muscle might not lie inconveniently low between the arm and thorax, as it would have done had the fibres which arise lowest from the sternum been inserted lowest in the arm; but this crossing does not make the tendon at all stronger, as is often said; nor can I see how it came to be thought that this tendon should want more strength in proportion than other tendons.

Deltoides arises exactly opposite to the insertion of the trapezius, from one third part of the clavicula, from the acromion and spine of the scapula, and is inserted tendinous near the middle of the os humeri, which bone it lifts directly upward. The outermost parts of this muscle, when the arm hangs down, lie below the centre of motion of the joint, and therefore can have no share in lifting the humerus up, till it is raised part of the way by the other part of this muscle, and the following muscle; and as the outer parts of this muscle begin to act, the following muscle acts with less advantage: and it seems to me, that the sole reason why this muscle is made of so many parts, is, that they may act independently; for it is demonstrable, that this muscle, when the whole of it acts, cannot raise the arm with so great advantage as a right lined muscle of the same magnitude would have done.

Supra-

Supraspinatus arifes from the dorfum fcapulæ above the fpine, and paffing between the two proceffes, is inferted into the upper part of the os humeri, which it helps to raife until it becomes parallel with the fpina fcapulæ.

The fupraspinatus, the deltoides, and coracobrachialis affift in all the motions of the humerus, except depreffion; it being neceffary that the arm fhould be raifed and fuftained, in order to move it to any fide.

Infraspinatus arifes from the dorfum fcapulæ below the fpine, and is inferted, wrapping over part of it, at the fide of the head of the os humeri; it turns the arm fupine and backward; for there is a prone and fupine rotatory motion of the humerus of near ninety degrees.

Teres minor is a fmall mufcle arifing below the former from the inferior cofta fcapulæ, and is inferted together with it. It affifts the former in turning the arm fupine, but pulls it more downwards.

Teres major arifes from the lower angle of the fcapula, and is inferted at the under part of the os humeri, about three fingers breadth from the head. This draws the os humeri toward the lower angle of the fcapula, and turns the arm prone and backward.

Latissimus dorsi arifes by a flat tendon from the fpinal proceffes of the feven or eight inferior vertebræ of the back, and thofe of the loins, ſacrum, and ilium; and growing fleſhy, after it has paſſed the extenſors of the trunk, receives another ſmall fleſhy beginning from the ninth, tenth, and eleventh ribs, and is inſerted into the os humeri, with the former. This turns the arm backward and prone. The tendon of this muſcle ſerves for a membrane to the extenſors of the back, and is connected to the tranſverſe proceſſes of the vertebræ lumborum.

SUBSCAPULARIS ariſes from the hollow ſide of the ſcapula, which it fills up, and is inſerted into the head of the os humeri, wrapping ſomewhat over it. This pulls the arm to the ſide and prone.

CORACOBRACHIALIS ariſes from the proceſſus coracoides ſcapulæ, in common with the origin of one head of the biceps, and is inſerted into the os humeri internally about its middle. This raiſes the arm, and turns it ſomewhat outward.

BICEPS CUBITI FLEXOR ariſes with two heads, that the fibres of this muſcle might not compreſs one another, one from the proceſſus coracoides ſcapulæ, in common with the coracobrachialis muſcle, and the other by a round tendon from the edge of the acetabulum ſcapulæ, which paſſing in a ſulcus of the os humeri, afterward becomes fleſhy, and joins the firſt head to be inſerted with it into the tubercle of the radius: and ſometimes this muſcle has a third head, which ariſes from the middle of the os humeri. This muſcle lifts up the humerus,

humerus, bends the cubit, and has as great a ſhare as any one muſcle in turning the cubit ſupine; the humerus being fixed by other muſcles, the whole force of this muſcle will be exerted upon the cubit; or the cubit being fixed by an extenſor, the whole force of it will be ſpent in raiſing the arm, and therefore ought to be always reckoned among thoſe that raiſe a weight at arms length. A puncture of the tendinous expanſion of this muſcle is ſuppoſed to be always attended with grievous pain and inflammation, and has, if we have not miſtaken the cauſe, often proved mortal; yet many eminent ſurgeons have given inſtances of larger tendons being cut and ſtiched, without any bad ſymptoms; and we have often ſeen them cut, torn, ulcerated, and mortified, without any more ſign of pain than in other parts. So that I cannot ſee what the great miſchief of pricking this tendinous faſcia is owing to, unleſs its lying ſo much upon the ſtretch, which may be wholly avoided by bending the elbow, and turning the cubit prone. Since I have conſidered this caſe, I have met with one who was thus injured by an injudicious blood-letter, who ordered the patient to keep her arm extended for fear of a contraction, and ſhe was not without the moſt violent pain for a whole fortnight; but upon bending the cubit, and turning the arm prone, ſhe grew preſently eaſy, and, in a few days, well. Nevertheleſs, I am perſuaded, that moſt of the accidents which

which are thought to be merely from blood-letting, are critical difcharges of fome difeafe, and from the puncture a fmall inflammation beginning, increafes and fuppurates. But however fingular I may be thought in this opinion, I can be fure I am difinterefted in it, having never had any ill accident follow blood-letting in my life.

BRACHIÆUS INTERNUS arifes from below the middle of the os humeri, and is inferted into a rough place of the ulna, immediately below the juncture. This alfo bends the cubit.

SUPINATOR RADII LONGUS arifes from the lower and outer part of the os humeri, and is inferted into the upper fide of the radius, near the carpus. This mufcle is not a fupinator but a bender of the cubit, and that with a longer lever than either of the two former mufcles, and is lefs concerned in turning the cubit fupine, than either the extenfors of the carpus, fingers, or thumb.

TRICEPS EXTENSOR CUBITI, commonly diftinguifhed into biceps and brachiæus externus. The firft of thefe heads arifes from the lower cofta of the fcapula near the acetabulum; the fecond from the outer and back part of the os humeri; the third, lower and more internal; and are inferted into the proceffus olecranon of the ulna. The firft of thefe heads draws the arm backward, with as long a lever as it extends the cubit.

ANCONÆUS arifes from the outward extuberance of

of the os humeri, and is inſerted into the upper part of the ulna: this is alſo an extenſor.

PALMARIS LONGUS ariſes ſmall from the inner extuberance of the os humeri, and from a ſhort belly ſoon becomes a tendon, which is connected to the ligamentum tranſverſale carpi, and expanded in the palm of the hand. This muſcle is often wanting, but the expanſion in the hand never; yet it being connected to the ligament of the carpus, it muſt bend the carpus, and cannot conſtrict the palm of the hand; and when it is wanting the flexor carpi radialis is larger.

PALMARIS BREVIS, OF CARO QUADRATA, ariſes obſcurely from the ligamentum tranſverſale carpi, and ſeems to be inſerted into the eighth bone of the carpus, and the metacarpal bone of the little finger. This helps to conſtrict the palm of the hand, and is very different in ſize in different bodies.

FLEXOR CARPI RADIALIS ariſes from the inner extuberance of the os humeri, and ſoon becoming a ſtrong tendon, paſſes through a chanel of the fifth bone of the carpus, and is inſerted into the metacarpal bone of the fore-finger. This not only bends the carpus upon the radius, but alſo the bones of the ſecond order upon thoſe of the firſt; which motion is nearly as much as that upon the radius.

FLEXOR CARPI ULNARIS ariſes from the ſame extuberance with the former, and a faſcia betwixt this muſcle and the tenſor ulnaris contiguous to the ulna,

ulna, and is inſerted by a ſhort tendon into the fourth bone of the carpus.

EXTENSORES CARPI RADIALES; the firſt ariſes from the os humeri, immediately below the ſupinator radii longus, and is inſerted into the metacarpal bone of the firſt finger; the ſecond ariſes immediately below this, from the outer extuberance of the os humeri, and is inſerted into the metacarpal bone of the ſecond finger. The firſt of theſe muſcles is a bender of the cubit, as well as an extenſor of the carpus, and its often acting with the benders of the cubit while the other is not in action, is the reaſon why it is ſo diſtinct from it.

EXTENSOR ULNARIS ariſes from the ſame extuberance with the former, and half the ulna below the anconeus muſcle; then becoming a tendon, runs in a ſmall ſinus at the bottom of the ulna, and is inſerted into the metacarpal bone of the little finger. See ULNA, p. 31, 32. The extenſors of the carpus being inſerted into the metacarpus, at once perform the motion between the bones of the carpus, and that between the carpus and radius. The flexor and tenſor ulnaris acting together turn the hand downward, the tenſor and flexor radialis upward.

PERFORATUS, or FLEXOR SECUNDI INTERNODII DIGITORUM ariſes from the inner tubercle of the os humeri, and from the upper part of the ulna, and the middle of the radius; then becoming four ſtrong tendons, paſſes under the ligamentum

tum transversale carpi, and is inserted into the beginning of the second bone of each finger.

PERFORANS, OF FLEXOR TERTII INTERNODII DIGITORUM, arises from half the ulna, and a great part of the ligament between the ulna and radius, then becoming four tendons, passes under the ligamentum transversale carpi, and through the tendons of the former muscle to their insertion into the third bone of each finger. The tendons of both these muscles are tied down to the fingers by a strong ligament. If these muscles had not passed one through the other, the perforatus, which is the lesser muscle, must have gone to the last joint where the stronger muscle is wanted; and, besides, the tendons of the second joints would have pressed those that bend the last, and not lain firmly upon them neither.

LUMBRICALES, OF FLEXORES PRIMI INTERNODII DIGITORUM, arise from the tendons of the last mentioned muscle, and are inserted laterally toward the thumb into the beginning of the first bone of each finger.

EXTENSOR DIGITORUM COMMUNIS arises from the outer extuberance of the os humeri, and passing under a ligament at the wrist, is divided into four tendons, which communicate upon the first joint, which keeps them from sliding off the joints of the fingers, where they are a little connected to the first bones, and afterward are inserted into the beginning of the second bone of each finger.

EXTENSOR AURICULARIS, or MINIMI DIGITI, is a portion of the laſt muſcle paſſing under the ligament in a diſtinct chanel.

EXTENSOR INDICIS ariſes from the middle of the ulna, and paſſing under the ligament of the carpus, is inſerted with the extenſor communis into the fore-finger. This muſcle extends the fore-finger ſingly. I have twice ſeen it wanting.

ABDUCTOR PRIMI DIGITI, INTEROSSEI, and ABDUCTOR MINIMI DIGITI, are eight muſcles, one for each ſide of each finger. Abductor primi digiti ariſes from the firſt bone of the thumb, and the ſide of the metacarpal bone of the firſt finger. The interoſſei are three pair, fitly divided into external and internal; the external ariſe from the metacarpal bones, whoſe ſpaces they fill up next the back of the hand; the internal ariſe from the ſame bones, in the inſide of the hand. Abductor minimi digiti ariſes from the tranſverſe ligament, and fourth bone of the carpus; theſe muſcles are inſerted, two into the firſt joint of each finger, and then paſſing obliquely over the tops of the fingers, are inſerted into their laſt bones; they bend the firſt joints, and extend the two laſt, as in holding a pen, and in playing upon ſome muſical inſtruments. The abductors of the fore and little fingers, with the ſecond and fifth interoſſei muſcles acting, the fingers are divaricated, and the other four acting bring them together, and theſe muſcles which divaricate the fingers,

fingers, being extenders of the ſecond and third joints, we never can divaricate them without extending them a little.

ADDUCTOR OSSIS METACARPI MINIMI DIGITI ariſes from the eighth bone and tranſverſe ligament of the carpus, and is inſerted into the metacarpal bone of the little finger, which it pulls toward the thumb to conſtrict the palm of the hand.

EXTENSOR PRIMI INTERNODII POLLICIS ariſes from the ulna below the anconeus muſcle, and the ligament between the ulna and radius; then becoming two, three, or four tendons, is inſerted into the fifth bone of the carpus, and firſt of the thumb. The firſt of theſe inſertions can only aſſiſt the bending of the wriſt upward, and in turning the arm ſupine.

EXTENSOR SECUNDI INTERNODII POLLICIS ariſes immediately below the former from the radius and tranſverſe ligament, and is inſerted by a few fibres into the ſecond bone of the thumb, but chiefly into the third.

EXTENSOR TERTII INTERNODII POLLICIS ariſes immediately below the laſt deſcribed, from the ulna and ligament, and paſſes over the radius nearer the ulna, to be inſerted at the third bone of the thumb. This extends the thumb more toward the ulna than the former muſcle, and is very much a ſupinator.

FLEXOR PRIMI ET SECUNDI OSSIS POLLICIS ariſes from the fifth bone and tranſverſe ligament

of

of the carpus, and from the beginnings of the two first metacarpal bones, and is inserted into the whole length of the first bone of the thumb, and tendinous into the beginning of the second; the sesamoid bones of the thumb in such bodies as have them, lie in this tendon, where it passes over the joint.

FLEXOR TERTII INTERNODII POLLICIS arises large from almost all the upper part of the radius, and becoming a round tendon, passes under the ligamentum transversale carpi, to be inserted into the third bone of the thumb. This muscle singly acting, draws the thumb towards the metacarpal bone of the little finger; but the last mentioned muscle acting with it, turns it toward the fore-finger.

ADDUCTOR POLLICIS arises from the carpus, and almost the whole length of the metacarpal bone of the long finger, and is inserted into the beginning of the second bone of the thumb. This muscle naturally enough divides into two, and might better be called a flexor than adductor.

ABDUCTOR POLLICIS arises from the fifth bone and ligamentum transversale of the carpus, and is inserted laterally into the beginning of the second bone of the thumb, to draw it toward the radius.

THE muscles which bend the thumb are much less than those which bend the fingers; nevertheless, the thumb is able to resist all the fingers, merely

merely from the advantages that arise from the thickness and shortness of the bones of the thumb, compared with those of the fingers; but then the quickness of motion in the fingers will exceed that of the thumb, as much as the fingers exceed the thumb in length, and their muscles those of the thumb in largeness.

SUPINATOR RADII BREVIS arises from the outer extuberance of the os humeri and upper part of the ulna, and running half round the radius, is inserted near its tubercle.

PRONATOR TERES arises from the inner apophysis of the os humeri, and upper and fore-part of the ulna, and is inserted tendinous into the radius below the former.

PRONATOR QUADRATUS arises from the lower edge of the ulna, near the carpus, and passing under the flexors of the fingers, is inserted into the radius.

THESE muscles are occasionally assisted in their actions by the muscles of the hands, the extensors assisting the supinators, and the flexors the pronators, and most of the extensors of the hand take a great part of their origin from the tendinous fascia that covers them.

MASTOIDEUS arises tendinous from the sternum near the clavicula, and by a separate fleshy portion from the clavicula, which soon unites with the other beginning, and is inserted to the outer part of the mamillary process of the temporal bone. It pulls that side of the head it is inserted

 into

into towards the ſternum, and turns the face toward the contrary ſhoulder. This, with its fellow, pull the head and neck toward the breaſt, and act with a much longer lever upon each lower vertebra, than they do upon the next above, and with more power upon any of thoſe joints than upon the head. This muſcle being inſerted into the head, beyond the centre of motion of the head with the firſt vertebra, has been ſuppoſed, by ſeveral anatomiſts, to pull the head backward; but the paſſing beyond ſignifies nothing to that purpoſe, unleſs a line going through its axis would paſs below the centre of motion: and it is the more to be wondered how this miſtake prevailed, if we conſider that this muſcle's being added to the extenſors of the head and neck, would make the force of that action a hundred times greater than that of the benders. And if this is not enough to convince, let any one lying on his back raiſe his head, and he will ſoon feel this muſcle in action; but bowing the head forward in an erect poſture will not ſhew this, unleſs ſome reſiſtance is made to the head, becauſe the centre of gravity of the head lying before the centre of motion, there needs no more than a relaxation of the extenſors, to bring the head forward in that poſture.

Rectus internus major ariſes from the anterior part of the tranſverſe proceſſes of the third, fourth, fifth, and ſixth cervical vertebræ; and paſſing over the two ſuperior, is inſerted into a rough-

 neſs

neſs of the occipital bone near the fore-part of the great foramen. This bends the head on the two firſt vertebræ of the neck.

RECTUS MINOR INTERNUS ariſes under the laſt muſcle, from the firſt vertebra, and is inſerted under it into the os occipitis. This bends the head on the firſt vertebra.

RECTUS LATERALIS ariſes from the anterior part of the tranſverſe proceſs of the firſt vertebra of the neck, and is inſerted into the os temporis and occipitis between the mamillary and ſtyloid proceſſes. This turns the head on one ſide.

SPLENIUS ariſes by a thin tendon from the ſpinal proceſſes of the five ſuperior vertebræ of the thorax, and the loweſt of the neck, and linea alba colli, and is inſerted into the os occipitis, the upper part of the mamillary proceſs of the temporal bone, and the tranſverſe proceſſes of the three ſuperior cervical vertebræ. This pulls the head and neck backward, and to the contrary ſide; but both of theſe acting together pull them directly backward.

COMPLEXUS ariſes from the tranſverſe proceſſes of the ſix or ſeven ſuperior vertebræ of the thorax, and ſix inferior of the neck, and is inſerted into the os occipitis, and back part of the os temporis; this laſt part is ſometimes diſtinct enough to be accounted another muſcle. It pulls the head and neck back.

RECTUS MAJOR POSTICUS arises from the spinal processes of the second vertebra of the neck, and is inserted broader into the os occipitis. It pulls the head back on the two first vertebræ.

RECTUS MINOR POSTICUS arises from the back part of the first vertebra of the neck, it having no spinal process, and is inserted below the former into the same bone, to pull the head back on the first vertebra.

OBLIQUUS SUPERIOR arises from the transverse process of the first vertebra, and is inserted into the os occipitis and back part of the os temporis, near the rectus major; either of these acting, assist the rectus lateralis on the same side; but both together pull the head back.

OBLIQUUS INFERIOR arises from the spinal process of the second vertebra of the neck, and is inserted into the transverse process of the first. This with its fellow alternately acting, turn the head with the first vertebra in a rotatory manner on the second, whose processus dentatus is the axis of this motion.

INTERSPINALES COLLI are three or four pair of muscles between the bifid processes of the cervical vertebræ, which they draw nearer each other when the neck is bent backward.

LONGUS COLLI arises laterally from the bodies of the four superior vertebræ of the thorax, and from the anterior part of the transverse processes of the five inferior vertebræ of the neck, and is inserted

ted into the fore-part of the first and second vertebræ of the neck, which it bends forward.

INTERTRANSVERSALES COLLI are portions of flesh between the transverse processes of the vertebræ of the neck, like the interspinales, but not so distinct; they draw these processes together.

SPINALIS COLLI arises from the transverse processes of the five superior vertebræ of the back, and is inserted into the spinal processes of the second, third, fourth, and fifth vertebræ of the neck. This pulls the neck backward.

TRANSVERSALIS COLLI arises from the oblique processes of the four inferior vertebræ of the neck, and is inserted into the spinal process of the second vertebra of the neck. This muscle is but a continuation of the transversalis or semispinalis dorsi.

THE muscles of the head and neck are most of them obliquely directed, which makes them perform the oblique motions, as well as extension and flexion; which is highly convenient in this case, because the joints moved by these muscles, being under the weight moved, it is necessary that the head should be kept steddy by the extensors, and flexors too, when any great weight is upon the head; and these muscles, from the obliquity of their directions, not only perform these two actions at once, but acting by pairs they move the head and neck steddily, in a diagonal direction, which strait muscles could not have done so well.

SCALENUS arises from the transverse processes of the second, third, fourth, fifth, and sixth cervical vertebræ. It is inserted, in three parts, into the two uppermost ribs, being thus divided for the transmission of the subclavian vessels. This muscle may bend the neck, but its chief use is to support the upper ribs, which is necessary to determine the contraction of the intercostal muscles that way, and a ligament could not have done this, because of the various positions that the neck and back are liable to.

SERRATUS SUPERIOR POSTICUS arises with a thin tendon, inseparable from the rhomboides, from the spinal process of the inferior cervical vertebra, and the three superior of the thorax, and is inserted into the second, third, and fourth ribs, immediately beyond their bendings; this, with the scalenus, sustains the upper ribs, that they might not be pulled downward by the depressors of the ribs in exspiration, as the lower ribs are upward in inspiration.

SERRATUS INFERIOR POSTICUS arises with a broad tendon, inseparable from that of the latissimus dorsi, from the spinal processes of the three superior vertebræ of the loins, and two inferior of the thorax, and is inserted into the tenth rib, but chiefly the ninth and eleventh: it pulls down the ribs in exspiration.

INTERCOSTALES are eleven pair on each side, in the interstices of the ribs; from their situations distin-

diſtinguiſhed into external and internal; they all ariſe from the under edge of each rib, and are inſerted into the upper edge of the rib below. The external are largeſt backward, having their firſt beginnings from the tranſverſe proceſſes of the vertebræ, like diſtinct muſcles, which ſome call levatores coſtarum. The internal run all from above obliquely backward; being thickeſt forward, and thinneſt toward the ſpine. Theſe are alſo continued betwixt the cartilages of the ſternum, with fibres perpendicular to the cartilages; and between the cartilages of the loweſt ribs, they are inſeparable from the obliquus aſcendens abdominis. Theſe muſcles, by drawing the ribs nearer to each other, pull them all upward, and dilate the thorax, they being ſuſtained at the top by the ſcalenus and ſerratus ſuperior poſticus. To theſe Mr. Cowper adds ſome fleſhy fibres, which run from one rib over a ſecond to a third, near the ſpine, which are levatores coſtarum.

Triangularis sterni ariſes internally from the cartilago enſiformis, and the lower edge of the os pectoris, and is inſerted into the end of the third, fourth, fifth, and ſixth ribs. This pulls the ribs to the bone of the ſternum, and thereby bends its cartilages in exſpiration.

Diaphragma ariſes on the right ſide by a proceſs from three lumbal vertebræ, and one of the thorax; and on the left, from the one ſuperior of the loins, and inferior of the thorax; this laſt part being leſs to give way to the great artery, and is inſerted into the lower part of the ſternum and the five inferior ribs. The middle of this muſcle is a flat tendon, from whence the fleſhy fibres begin and are diſtributed, like radii, from a centre to a circumference. When this muſcle acts alone, it conſtricts the thorax, and pulls the ribs downward, and approaches toward a plane; which action is generally performed to promote the ejection of the fæces. In large inſpirations, when the intercoſtals lift up the ribs to widen the thorax, this muſcle acts enough to bring itſelf toward a plane, without overcoming the force of the intercoſtals, by which means the breaſt is at once widened and lengthened: when it acts with the abdominal muſcles, it draws the ribs nearer together, and conſtricts the thorax, and the ſuperior force of the abdominal muſcles thruſting the parts of the lower belly againſt it, it becomes at the ſame time convex upward, and ſhortens the thorax, which occaſions the largeſt exſpirations; or acting alternately with the abdominal muſcles only, a more moderate inſpiration and exſpiration is made by ſhortening and lengthening the thorax only, which is what we chiefly do when lying down; or acting alternately with the intercoſtals only, a moderate exſpiration and inſpiration is cauſed, by the widening and narrowing the breaſt, which is what we are moſt prone to in an erect poſition, the muſcles of the abdomen at ſuch times being employed in ſupporting the parts con-

tained

tained in the abdomen. And though theſe motions of the ribs require at any one time but very little force, the air within the thorax balancing that without; yet that theſe muſcles, whoſe motions are eſſential to life, may be never weary, the inſpirators in moſt men have force ſufficient to raiſe mercury in a tube four or five and twenty inches in an erect poſture, and the exſpirators ſix or ſeven; the firſt of which will require about four thouſand pound force in moſt men, and the other proportional. But I imagine, that lying down, theſe proportions will differ by the weight of the parts contained in the abdomen. In all the bodies I have diſſected, I have found the diaphragm convex upward, which gave me occaſion to think, that all animals died in exſpiration; till the forementioned experiment diſcovered, that the muſcles of inſpiration were ſtronger than thoſe of exſpiration; which led me to make the following experiment. I cut the wind-pipe of a dog, and having a ſtring ready fixed, I put a cork into it, and tied it faſt inſtantly, after inſpiration; upon which I obſerved, that the diaphragm, and the other muſcles of inſpiration and exſpiration, were alternately contracted and diſtended for ſome time; but when he was dead, the abdominal muſcles were in a ſtate of contraction, the ribs were elevated to dilate the thorax, and the diaphragm was convex upward. This experiment alſo ſhews, that the diaphragm is not a muſcle of equal force either to the depreſſors or elevators of the

the ribs, it neither hindering the elevators from raiſing the breaſt; nor the depreſſors from thruſting it upward, by compreſſing the parts contained in the abdomen, though the breaſt was full of air.

SACER SACROLUMBALIS, LONGISSIMUS DORSI, and SEMISPINALIS, are all that portion of fleſh betwixt the os ſacrum and the neck, which, ſeeing there is no membrane to diſtinguiſh it into ſeveral muſcles, and that it is all employed in the ſame actions, I ſhall give it the name of extenſor dorſi et lumborum, and deſcribe it all as one muſcle.

EXTENSOR DORSI ET LUMBORUM ariſes from the upper part of the os ſacrum, the ſpine of the os ilium, the back parts of the lowermoſt vertebræ of the loins, and remarkably from thoſe ſtrong tendons which appear on their outſides. That part of this muſcle, which is known by the name of ſacrolumbalis, is inſerted into all the ribs near their articulations, with the tranſverſe proceſſes of the vertebræ, and into the tranſverſe proceſs of the laſt vertebra of the neck; beſides, as this paſſes over the ribs, it receives an origin from every rib, in a manner that cannot well be deſcribed. The portions of this muſcle, which ariſe from the ribs, and are inſerted into the other ribs above, will neceſſarily draw the back part of the ribs nearer together, which muſt always be done as the back extends, and independent of other actions of the thorax. The next portion of this muſcle, called longiſſimus dorſi,

is

is inſerted into all the tranſverſe proceſſes of the vertebræ of the back, and partly into the ribs, and the uppermoſt tranſverſe proceſſes of the vertebræ of the loins; and the upper end of it is neither very diſtinct from the complexus of the head, nor ſpinalis of the neck. The reſt of this muſcle, known by the names of ſemiſpinalis, ſacer, etc. ariſes alſo from all the tranſverſe and oblique proceſſes of the loins and back; every portion, except the lowermoſt, paſſing over five joints, is inſerted into the ſpinal proceſs of the ſixth vertebra above its origin, all the way up the back, and at the neck commences tranſverſalis colli. This paſſing of each portion of a muſcle over a few joints, diſtributes their force equally enough among all theſe joints, without the fibres being directed more obliquely than thoſe of penniform muſcles; but the neck and loins not having ſufficient proviſion of this ſort, there are ſmall muſcles between their proceſſes, which, though they are of little importance for the motions of thoſe parts, yet are ſufficient to diſtribute the force of larger muſcles equally among thoſe joints; and beſides the uſes of the extenſor dorſi et lumborum, which its name implies, it and its fellow alternately raiſe the hips in walking, which any one may feel by laying his hand upon his back.

QUADRATUS LUMBORUM ariſes from the upper part of the ſpine of the ilium, and is inſerted into all the tranſverſe proceſſes of the four upper-

moſt

moſt lumbal vertebræ. This, with its fellow, acting alternately, aſſiſt the laſt mentioned muſcle in raiſing the oſſa innominata in progreſſion : or each acting ſingly, while the lower limbs are not moved, inclines the body to one ſide.

INTERTRANSVERSALES LUMBORUM are ſmall muſcles ſeated between all the tranſverſe proceſſes of the vertebræ lumborum, to bring them nearer together.

PSOAS PARVUS ariſes laterally from the body of the firſt lumbal vertebra, and the loweſt of the back, and ſoon becoming a ſmall tendon, is inſerted into the os pubis, near the ilium. It either aſſiſts in bending the loins forward, or raiſing the os innominatum in progreſſive motions. This muſcle is often wanting.

PSOAS MAGNUS ariſes laterally from the bodies and tranſverſe proceſſes of the four ſuperior vertebræ of the loins, and the laſt of the back, and is inſerted, with the following muſcle, into the leſſer trochanter. This bends the thigh, and when the pſoas parvus is wanting, this is larger.

ILIACUS INTERNUS ariſes from the concave part of the ilium, and from its lower edge, and paſſing over the ilium, near the os pubis, joins the former muſcle, and is inſerted with it, to be employed in the ſame action.

PECTINEUS ariſes from the os pubis or pectinis, near the joining of that bone with its fellow, and is inſerted into the linea aſpera of the thigh bone,

four

four fingers breadth below the leſſer trochanter. This bends the thigh, and turns the toes outward.

TRICEPS FEMORIS. The two leſſer heads of this muſcle ariſe under the pectineus, and the third from the inferior edges and back part of the os pubis and iſchium, and is inſerted into the whole length of the linea aſpera and the inner apophyſis of the os femoris. This alſo bends the thigh, and turns the toes outward. When the thigh bone is moved in a plane, which cuts at right angles a plane that paſſes through the axis of either head of the laſt muſcle, that head riſing lower than the centre of motion of the hip joint, it will either aſſiſt the flexors or extenſors, and that moſt when the bone has been moved moſt backward or forward; and as either of theſe heads lie more or leſs out of the ſaid plane, they will give greater aſſiſtance to that motion which is made on the ſide of the ſaid plane, contrary to their ſituation, and leſs on the ſame ſide. This mechaniſm is frequently made uſe of to make one muſcle ſerve different actions; but I have only explained it in this inſtance, becauſe it is the moſt conſiderable one that I know.

GLUTEUS MAXIMUS ariſes from the back part of the ſpine of the ilium, and the dorſum ilii, and ſide of the os coccygis and ſacrum, and a ligament extended between theſe bones, and from a thin faſcia, ſpread over that part of the following muſcle which this does not cover, and is inſerted by a ſtrong a ſtrong tendon into the upper part of the linea aſpera of the thigh bone, and alſo into the flat tendon of the faſcialis muſcle, which inſertion into, or connection with, that tendon raiſes this muſcle farther from the centre of motion, and increaſes its ſtrength. This extends the thigh, and both theſe together being contracted, occaſionally aſſiſt the levatores ani in ſupporting the anus. The breadth of the origin and inſertion of this muſcle is very obſervable, for by that means, though it is the largeſt muſcle in the body, it is nevertheleſs rightlined, without one fibre compreſſing another any more than in penniform muſcles.

Gluteus medius ariſes from all the anterior part of the ſpina and dorſum ilii, and under part of the laſt mentioned muſcle, and is inſerted into the upper part of the great trochanter of the thigh bone. This extends the thigh outward.

Gluteus minimus ariſes intirely under the former, from the dorſum ilii, and is inſerted into the upper and anterior part of the great trochanter and neck of the thigh bone to extend the thigh.

Pyriformis ariſes internally from the inſide of the os ſacrum, and growing, in more than half its progreſs, into a round tendon, is inſerted into the upper part of the ſinus, at the root of the great trochanter. This aſſiſts ſomewhat in extending the thigh, but more in turning it outward.

Quadratus femoris ariſes from the obtuſe proceſs of the iſchium, and is inſerted into the upper

per part of the linea aſpera of the thigh bone, between the two trochanters. This draws the thigh inward, and directs the toes outward.

Obturator internus or marsupialis ariſes generally from a ſtrong membrane, or ligament, which fills up the hole of the os innominatum, and from the circumambient bone; thence paſſing over a chanel in the iſchium, betwixt its two proceſſes, it receives from them two other portions, which are a ſort of marſupium, and is inſerted into the ſinus of the great trochanter. This turns the thigh outward.

Obturator externus ariſes oppoſite to the former, from the outſide of the os innominatum, and is inſerted into the ſinus of the great trochanter. This alſo turns the thigh outward. Theſe four laſt mentioned muſcles acting with the extenſors, prevent their turning the toes inward, and in ſtepping forwards are continually acting to turn the toes outwards; for though the toes are placed perpendicular to the front of the body, in taking a long ſtep, theſe muſcles bring them perpendicular to the ſide of the body; and as theſe direct, the ſame extenſors will turn the thigh either outward or backward, with their full force.

Fascialis, or membranosus, ariſes from the fore-part of the ſpine of the ilium, and in about five inches progreſs becomes a flat tendon, or faſcia, which is joined by a conſiderable detachment from the tendon of the gluteus maximus, and from the linea

linea aſpera of the thigh bone, and then covering in an eſpecial manner the vaſtus externus, is inſerted at the top of the tibia and fibula, and then proceeds to join the faſcia, which covers the upper part of the muſcles ſituate on the outſide of the tibia, and from which a great part of the fibres of thoſe muſcles ariſe. About the middle of the leg it grows looſe, and is ſo continued to the top of the foot, being connected there and at the lower part of the leg, to the ligaments which tie down the tendons. This tendon, where it covers the vaſtus externus, receives additional tranſverſe fibres, which run round the thigh, but are moſt conſpicuous on the outſide. This draws the thigh outward, and paſſing over the knee forwarder than its axis of motion, it will help to extend that joint.

Gracilis ariſes from the os pubis, cloſe to the penis, and is inſerted into the tibia, four or five fingers breadth below the knee. This draws the thigh inward, and paſſing over the knee, behind its axis of motion, it will help to bend it.

Sartorius ariſes from the fore-part of the ſpine of the ilium, and thence deſcending obliquely to the inſide of the tibia, is there inſerted four or five fingers breadth below the joint. This at once helps to bend both the thigh and leg, particularly the thigh, at very long levers; it directly helps to lift up the leg in walking up ſtairs, or laying the legs acroſs, like taylors.

Semi-

Semitendinosus arises from the obtuse process of the ischium, and growing a round tendon in somewhat more than half its progress, is inserted near the former muscles into the tibia: it helps to extend the thigh and bend the tibia.

Semimembranosus arises by a flat tendon like a membrane from the obtuse process of the ischium, and being continued tendinous betwixt the bellies of the last-mentioned and following muscles, and then growing fleshy, becomes again tendinous above the joint, and is inserted nearer the joint than the former muscle for the same use.

These two make the internal hamstring, and arising and inserting so near together, they might have been one muscle, but their fibres would have been near twice as long, which would have given a motion near twice as quick, but not so strong, unless it had been inserted at a distance from the joint it moves proportionable to its length, which could not well be; therefore they are made two muscles of a number of fibres nearly equal to what one could have been, and are inserted at distances from the axis of motion of the knee, proportional to the different lengths of their fibres in the directions of their axes.

Biceps tibiæ, the first head arises in common with the two preceding muscles, from the obtuse process of the ischium; the second from the lower part of the linea aspera of the thigh bone. This soon joins the former, and is inserted with it into the upper part of the fibula to bend the leg, and the first head also extends the thigh. The tendon of this muscle makes the external hamstring, when the knee is bent; and when we sit down, the biceps will turn the leg and toes outward, and the semitendinosus and semimembranosus will turn them inward.

Popliteus arises from the outer apophysis of the os femoris, and thence running obliquely inward, is inserted into the tibia immediately below its head. This assists the flexors, and draws the tibia toward the outer apophysis of the thigh bone.

Rectus tibiæ arises with a tendon from the upper part of the acetabulum of the os innominatum, and by another tendon, which is a sort of ligament to this, from a processus innominatus of the ilium below its spine forward, and is inserted, together with the three following muscles, into the patella. It bends the thigh, and extends the tibia.

Vastus externus arises from the anterior part of the great trochanter and upper part of the linea aspera of the thigh bone, and is inserted into the upper and external part of the patella. It extends the tibia.

Vastus internus arises from the inner and lower part of the linea aspera, and is inserted into the upper and inner part of the patella, to extend the tibia; and the fibres of this muscle being oblique, it keeps the patella in its place, the other muscles lying in the direction of the os femoris

which

which makes an obtuſe angle with the tibia, they would alone be liable to draw the patella outward. This contrivance is moſt obvious in thoſe whoſe knees bend moſt inward.

CRUREUS ariſes between the two laſt, below the rectus, from all the convex part of the os femoris, and is inſerted in like manner into the patella; the patella being tied down by a ſtrong ligament to the tibia. Theſe three laſt muſcles extend the tibia only, and might very properly be called extenſor tibiæ triceps.

GASTEROCNEMIUS ariſes by two ſmall beginnings above the back part of the apophyſis of the os femoris, which ſoon becoming large bellies unite, and then become a flat tendon which joins the following muſcles to be inſerted into the os calcis. The two parts of this muſcle are by ſome writers diſtinguiſhed into two muſcles. Its uſe is to extend the tarſus and bend the knee.

PLANTARIS ariſes under the outer beginning of the laſt named muſcle, from the external apophyſis of the os femoris, and ſoon becoming a ſmall tendon, is ſo continued betwixt the foregoing and ſubſequent muſcles, and is inſerted with them. It bends the knee, and extends the tarſus. Authors derive the tendinous expanſion on the bottom of the foot from the tendon of this muſcle; but ſeeing the expanſion is much more than this tendon could make, and that this tendon can he traced no farther than the os calcis, and that the expanſion is as large when the muſcle is wanting, which is not ſeldom, I cannot be of that opinion.

GASTEROCNEMIUS INTERNUS ariſes from the upper part of the tibia, and one third of the fibula, below the popliteus, and is inſerted with the two foregoing muſcles by a ſtrong tendon into the upper and back part of the os calcis. This muſcle only extends the tarſus.

TIBIALIS ANTICUS ariſes from the upper and exterior part of the tibia, and is inſerted laterally into the os cuneiforme majus of the tarſus, and by a ſmall portion of its tendon into the metacarpal bone of the great toe. This bends and turns the tarſus inward.

TIBIALIS POSTICUS ariſes firſt by a ſmall beginning from the upper part of the tibia between that bone and the fibula then paſſing between the bones through a perforation in the tranſverſe ligament which connects thoſe bones, it takes other beginnings from the upper and middle part of the tibia, and from the middle of the fibula, and the ligament betwixt the tibia and fibula; then growing a round tendon, paſſes under the inner ancle, and is inſerted into the lower part of the os naviculare, and into the os cuneiforme majus. This extends and turns inward the tarſus.

PERONEUS LONGUS ariſes from the upper and outer part of the fibula, and growing a tendon toward the lower part of this bone, passes under the outer ancle, and the muscles situated on the bottom of the foot, and is inserted into the beginning of the metatarsal bone of the great toe, and the os cuneiforme next that bone. This turns the tarsus outward, and directs the force of the other extensors of the tarsus toward the ball of the great toe.

Peroneus brevis arises from the middle of the fibula, under a part of the former, and growing tendinous, passes under the outer ancle, and is inserted into the beginning of the upper part of the os metatarsi of the little toe, and sometimes bestows a small tendon on the little toe. Its use is to extend the tarsus, and turn it outward.

These two last muscles riding over the lower end of the fibula, are often the cause of a sprain in the outer ancle, when they are vehemently exerted to save a fall.

Extensor pollicis longus arises from the upper and middle part of the fibula and the ligamentum transversale, and soon becoming a strong tendon, is inserted into the last bone of the great toe. This also bends the tarsus with a much longer lever than it extends the toe.

Extensor pollicis brevis arises from the fore part of the os calcis, and is inserted into the same place with the former.

Flexor pollicis longus arises from the fibula, opposite to the extensor longus, and then paſſing under the inner ancle, is inſerted into the under ſide of the laſt bone of the great toe. This extends the tarſus at a longer lever than it bends the toe.

FLEXOR BREVIS and ADDUCTOR POLLICIS are the ſame muſcle, ariſing from the two leſſer oſſa cuneiformia and os cuboides and calcis. They are inſerted into the oſſa ſeſamoidea, which are tied by a ligament to the firſt bone of the great toe, reckoning only two bones to the great toe. Theſe muſcles bend the great toe.

ABDUCTOR POLLICIS ariſes pretty largely from the inner and back part of the os calcis, and by a ſmaller beginning from the os naviculare; thence paſſing forward contiguous to the os cuneiforme majus, paſſes by the external ſeſamoid bone of the great toe to its inſertion into the firſt bone of the great toe. This muſcle is leſs an abductor than a flexor pollicis pedis; it alſo very much helps to conſtrict the foot lengthways.

TRANSVERSALIS PEDIS ariſes from the lower end of the metatarſal bone of the toe next the leaſt, and is inſerted into the internal ſeſamoid bone. This truly is an adductor of the great toe, and helps to keep the conſtrictor of the bottom of the foot.

EXTENSOR DIGITORUM PEDIS LONGUS ariſes acute from the upper part of the tibia, and from the upper and middle part of the fibula and ligament between theſe bones; then dividing into five tendons, four of them are inſerted into the ſecond

bone

bone of each leſſer toe, and the fifth into the beginning of the metatarſal bone of the leaſt toe, and ſometimes by a ſmall tendon alſo into the little toe. This laſt portion for the moſt part is ſeparate from its beginning, and may be accounted a diſtinct muſcle. The four firſt tendons only of this muſcle extend the toes, but all five bend the tarſus, and that with a longer lever than any of them bend a toe.

Extensor digitorum brevis, ariſes together with the extenſor pollicis brevis, from the os calvis, and dividing into three ſmall tendons is inſerted into the ſecond joint of the three toes next the great one. The long extenſors of the toes ſerve not only to extend them, but alſo contribute to the bending of the ancle, which motions are uſually performed together in progreſſion; but the ſhort extenſors ariſing below the ancle, extend the toes only; and when the long extenſors are employed for that action only, the extenſors of the tarſus muſt act at the ſame time, to prevent the bending of the ancle. This is the reaſon why the toes have need, though their motions are leſs, of more extenſors than the fingers.

Flexor brevis or perforatus ariſes from the under and back part of the os calcis, thence paſſing toward the four leſſer toes, divides into four tendons, which are inſerted into the beginning of the ſecond bone of each of the leſſer toes. Theſe tendons are divided to let through the tendons of the following muſcles.

Flexor longus or perforans ariſes from the back part of the tibia, above the inſertion of the popliteus, and part of the fibula; thence deſcending under the os calcis to the bottom of the foot, there becomes tendinous, often croſſes, and, in moſt bodies, communicates with the flexor longus pollicis pedis; then it divides into four tendons, which paſs through thoſe of the flexor brevis, and are inſerted into the third bone of the four leſſer toes. This muſcle alſo extends the tarſus. The ſecond beginning of this muſcle ariſes from the os calcis, and joins the tendons where they divide. This portion only bends the toes; and ſeeing the flexor longus of the toes will, when it acts alone, extend the tarſus as well as bend the toes, this portion, like the ſhort extenſors of the toes, ſeems purpoſely contrived to bend the toes alone.

Lumbricales ariſe from the tendons of the perforans, and are inſerted into the firſt bone of each of the leſſer toes which they bend.

Abductor minimi digiti pedis ariſes by the perforatus from the os calcis, and being part of it inſerted into the metacarpal bone of the leaſt toe, it receives another beginning from the os cuboides, and is inſerted into the firſt bone of the leaſt toe, which it bends and pulls outward, and very much helps to conſtrict the bottom of the foot.

Abductor secundus minimi digiti ariſes under the former muſcle from the metatarſal bone, and is inſerted into the little toe.

Inter-

Interossei are seven muscles which lie like those of the hands, and arise like them from the metatarsal bones, and are inserted like them into the last joints of the four lesser toes; and being in their progress attached to the tendons, which extend the second joints of the toes, they will extend both these joints. These muscles may be fitly divided into external and internal; the internal also bend the first joints, as do all the interossei in the hand, but here the outer ones extend the first joints; and if we consider that the first of these muscles is analogous to the abductor indicis of the hand, and that the abductor minimi is alike in both, we find that the muscles to move the fingers and lesser toes sideways are alike in number, though this motion of the toes is in a manner lost from the use of shoes. The muscles that bend or extend the last joints of the toes will also move the second and first, and those that move the second will also move the first, as they do in the fingers.

TAB. XI.

TAB. XI.

1 Musculus frontalis.
2 Temporalis.
3 Orbicularis.
4 The parotid gland, with its duct, which passes through the buccinator.
5 Mastoideus.
6 Zygomaticus.
7 Elevator labii superioris proprius.
8 Elevator labiorum communis.
9 Depressor labiorum communis.
10 Sphincter oris.
11 Depressor labii inferioris proprius.
12 Buccinator.
13 Sterno-hyoidei.
14 Coraco-hyoideus.
15 Mastoideus.
16 Trapezius.
17 Pectoralis.
18 Deltoides.

TAB. XII.

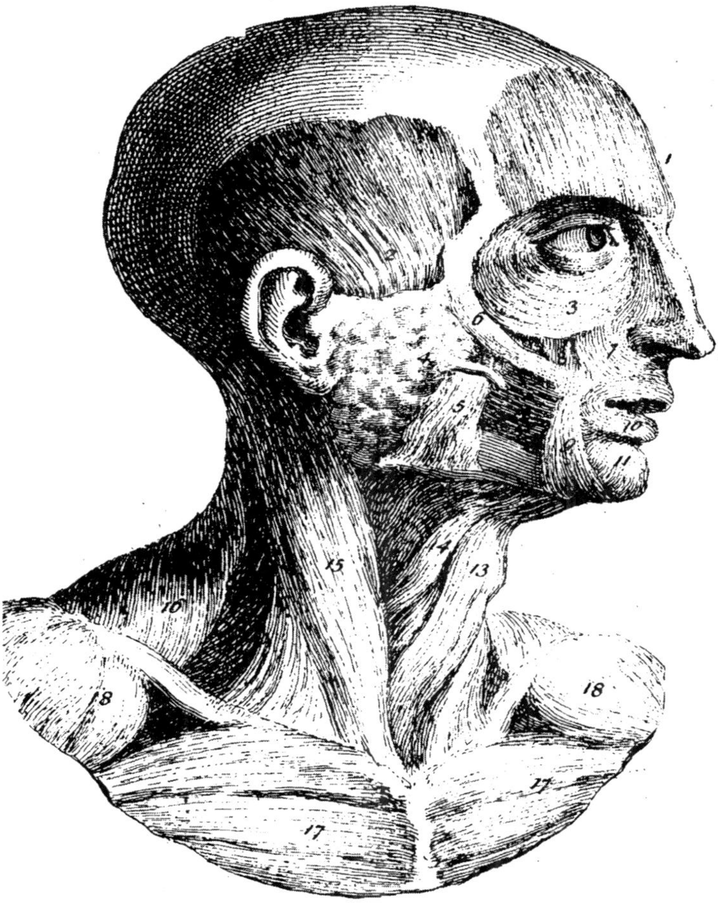

TAB. XII.

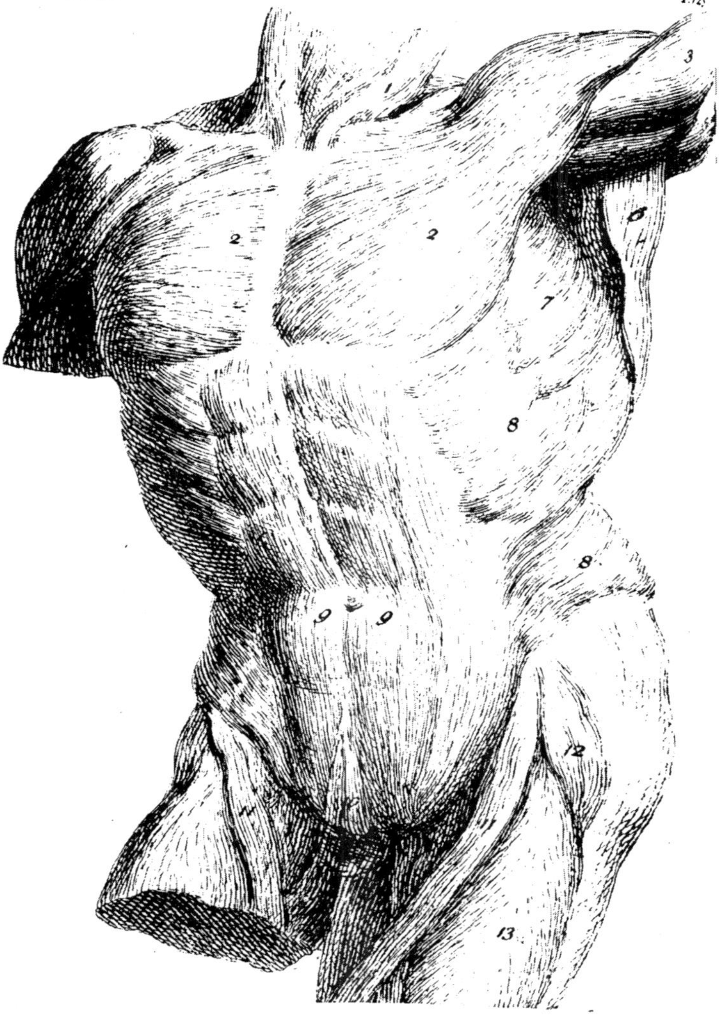

TAB. XII.

1 Mufculus maftoideus.
2 Pectoralis.
3 Biceps flexor cubiti.
4 Coraco-brachialis.
5 Triceps extenfor cubiti.
6 Latiffimus dorfi.
7 Seratus major anticus.
8 Obliquus defcendens abdominis.
9 Rectus abdominis.
10 Pyramidalis.
11 Sartorius.
12 Fafcialis.
13 Rectus femoris.

TAB. XIII.

TAB. XIII.

1 Trapezius.
2 Deltoides.
3 Infra ſpinatus ſcapulæ.
4 Teres major.
5 Rhomboides.
6 Latiſſimus dorſi.
7 Glutæi.
8 Obliquus deſcendens abdominis.

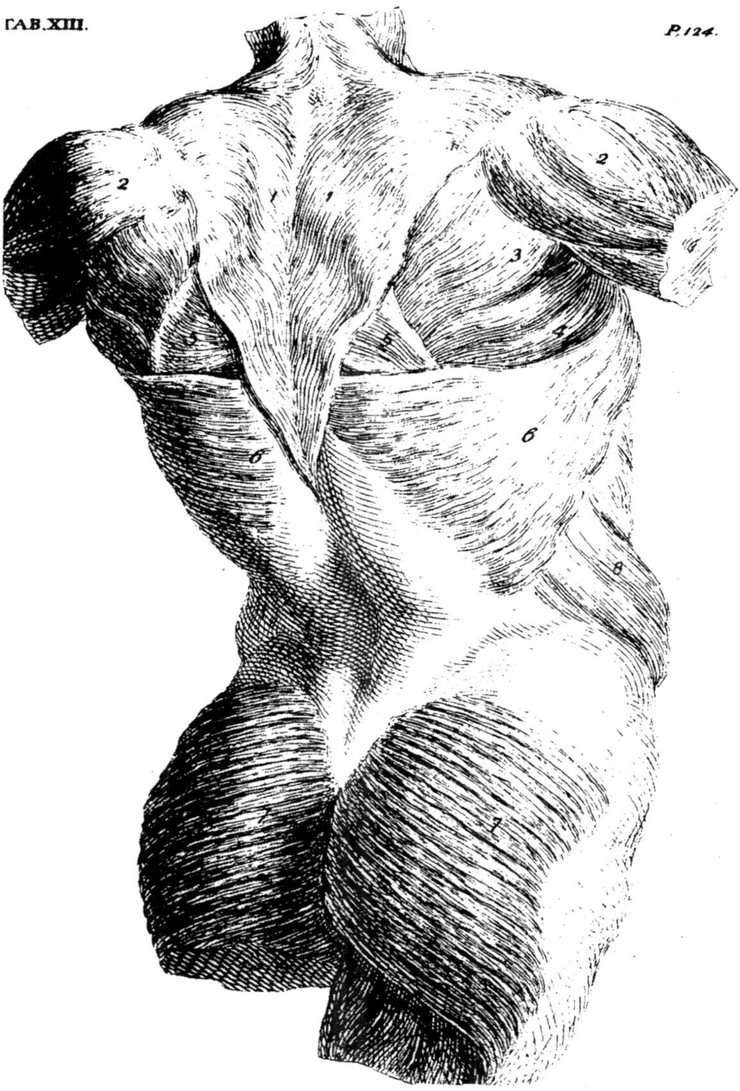
1
1
2
2
3
4
5
5
6
6
7
8

TAB. XIV.

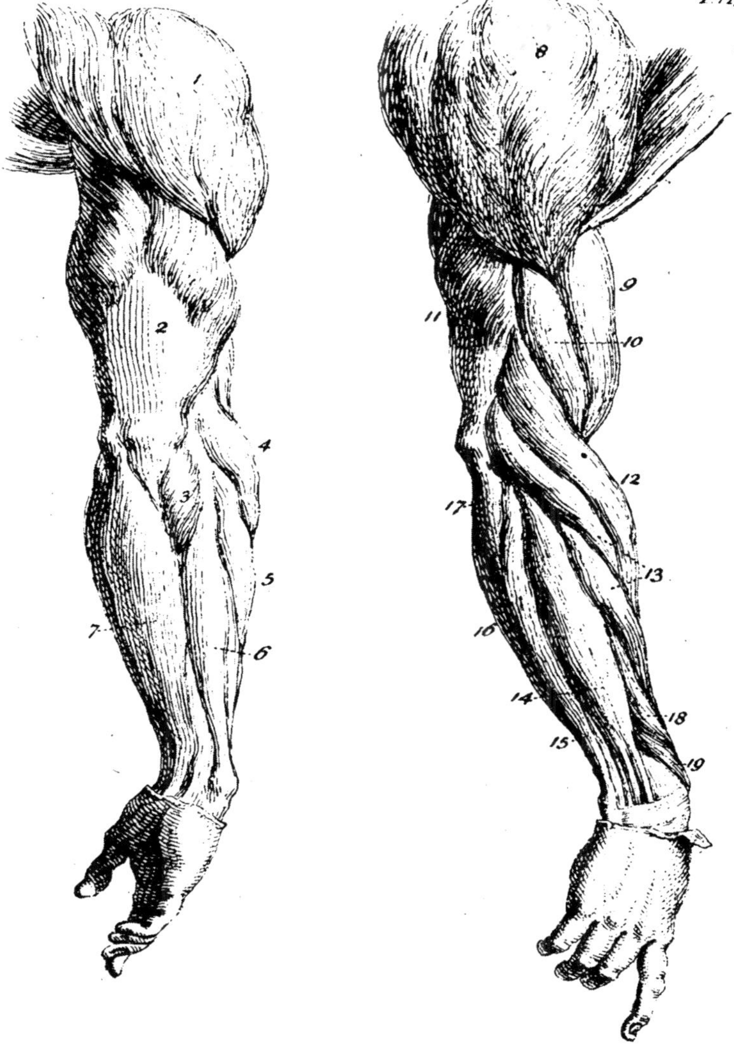

TAB. XIV.

1 Muſculus deltoides.
2 Triceps extenſor cubiti.
3 Anconæus.
4 Extenſor carpi radialis primus.
5 Extenſor carpi radialis ſecundus.
6 Extenſor carpi ulnaris.
7 Flexor carpi ulnaris.
8 Deltoides.
9 Biceps flexor cubiti.
10 Brachiæus internus.
11 Triceps extenſor cubiti.
12 Supinator radii longus.
13 Extenſores carpi radiales.
14 Extenſor communis digitorum.
15 Extenſor carpi ulnaris.
16 Flexor carpi ulnaris.
17 Anconæus.
18 Extenſor pollicis primus.
19 Extenſor pollicis ſecundus.

TAB. XV.

1 Musculus deltoides.
2 Pectoralis.
3 Biceps flexor cubiti.
4 Triceps extensor cubiti.
5 The fascia tendinosa of the biceps muscle.
6 Supinator radii longus.
7 Flexor carpi radialis.
8 Glutæus.
9 Vastus externus.
10 Biceps femoris.
11 Semitendinosus.
12 Semimembranosus.
13 Gastrocnemius.
14 Solæus.

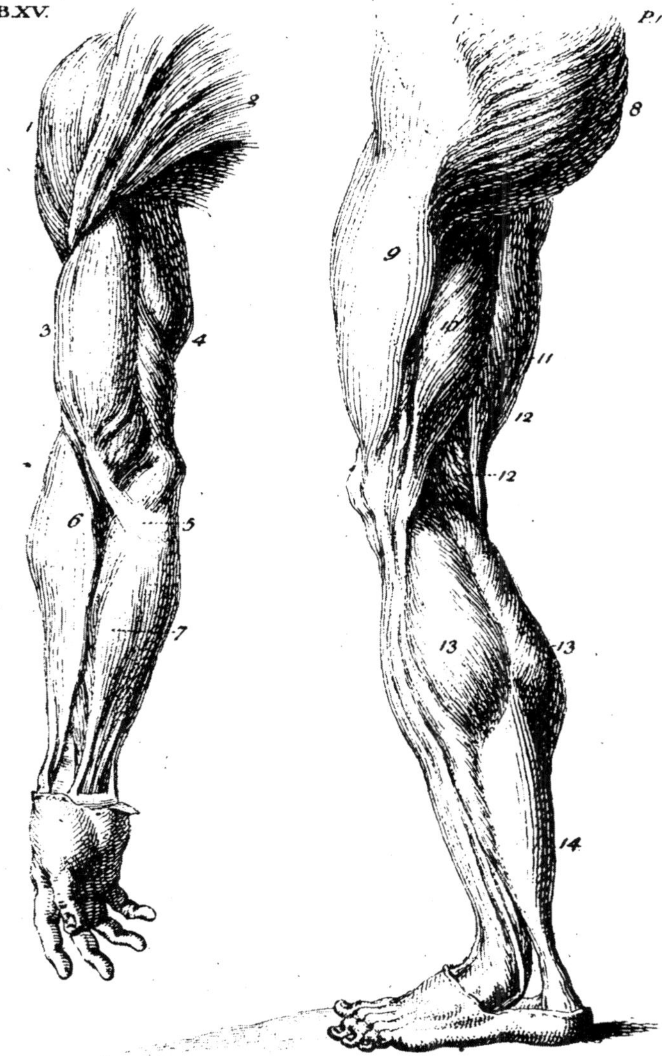
1
2
3
4
5
6
7
8
9
10
11
12
12
13
13
14

XVI. P.127

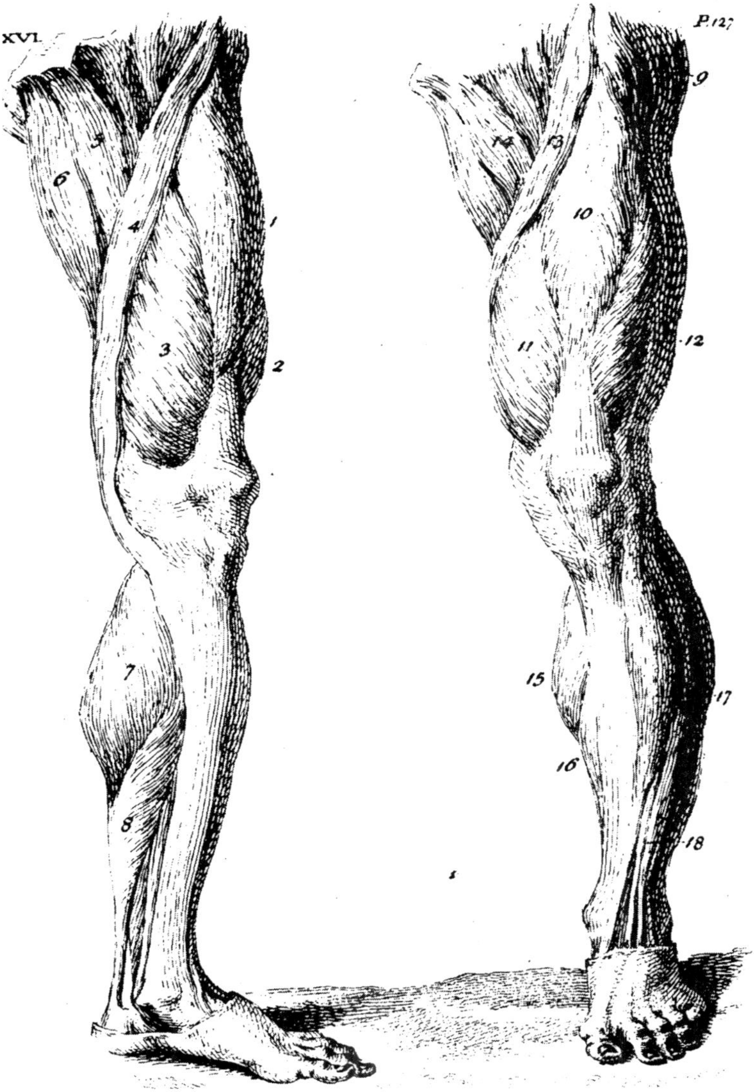

TAB. XVI.

1 Musculus rectus femoris.
2 Vastus externus.
3 Vastus internus.
4 Sartorius.
5 Pectinæus.
6 The large head of the triceps.
7 Gastrocnemius.
8 Solæus.
9 Membranosus.
10 Rectus femoris.
11 Vastus internus.
12 Vastus externus.
13 Sartorius.
14 Pectinæus.
15 Gastrocnemius.
16 Solæus.
17 Tibialis anticus.
18 Extensores digitorum.

T A B. XVII.

1 Mufculus abductor pollicis.
2 Adductor pollicis.
3 Flexor brevis.
4 Quadratus feu palmaris brevis.
5 The ftrong ligament of the carpus that binds down the tendons of the flexors of the fingers.
6 Abductor minimi digiti.
7 A probe under the tendons of the perforatus.
8 A probe under the tendons of the perforans.
9 Lumbricales.
10 Perforatus.
11 Flexor carpi radialis.
12 Flexor carpi ulnaris.

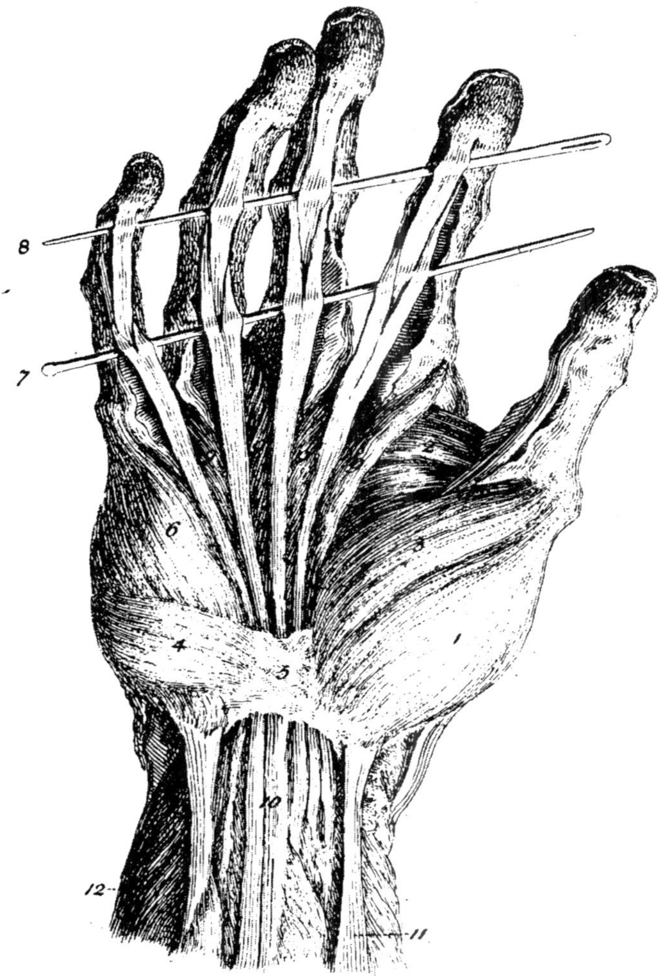
8
7
6
4
5
1
2
3
10
12
11

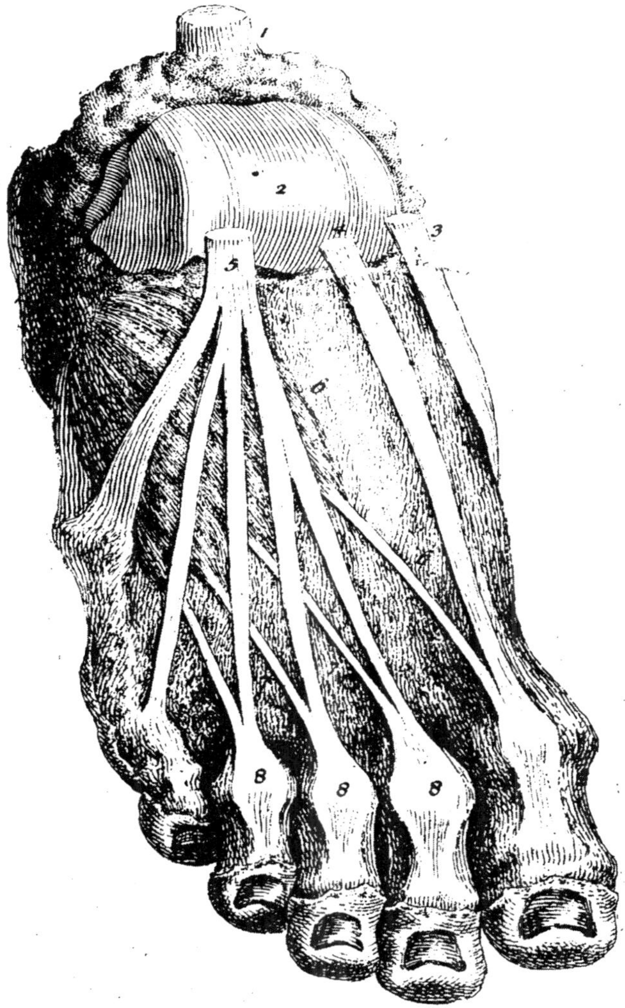
1
2
3
4
5
6
8
8
8

TAB. XVIII.

1 Tendo achilles.
2 That part of the aſtragalus which articulates with the tibia.
3 The tendon of the tibialis anticus.
4 The tendon of the extenſor pollicis pedis longus.
5 The tendons of the extenſor digitorum communis.
6 Extenſor pollicis pedis brevis.
7 Extenſor digitorum brevis.
8 The union of the tendons of the extenſor longus and the extenſor brevis.

TAB. XIX.

1 Musculus triceps extensor cubiti.
2 Deltoides.
3 Teres major.
4 Latissimus dorsi.
5 Pectoralis.
6 Obliquus descendens abdominis.
7 Rectus abdominis.
8 Sartorius.
9 Rectus femoris
10 Vastus externus.
11 Vastus internus.
12 Gastrocnemius.
13 Solæus.
14 Tibialis anticus.

TAB. XX.

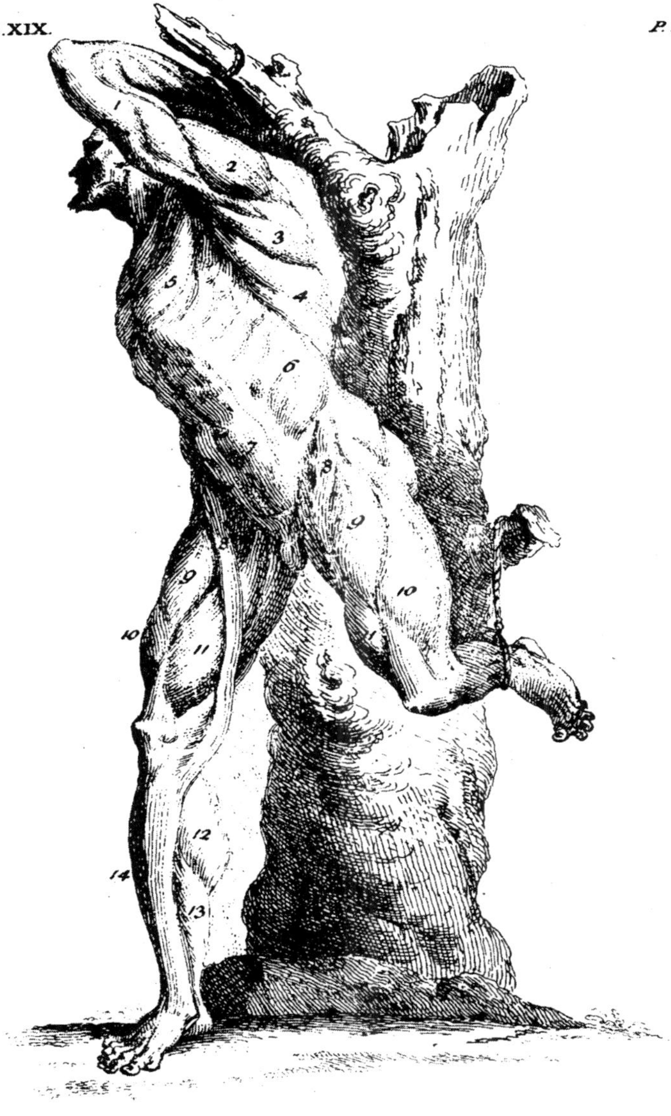
1
2
3
4
5
6
7
8
9
10
11
9
10
11
12
13
14

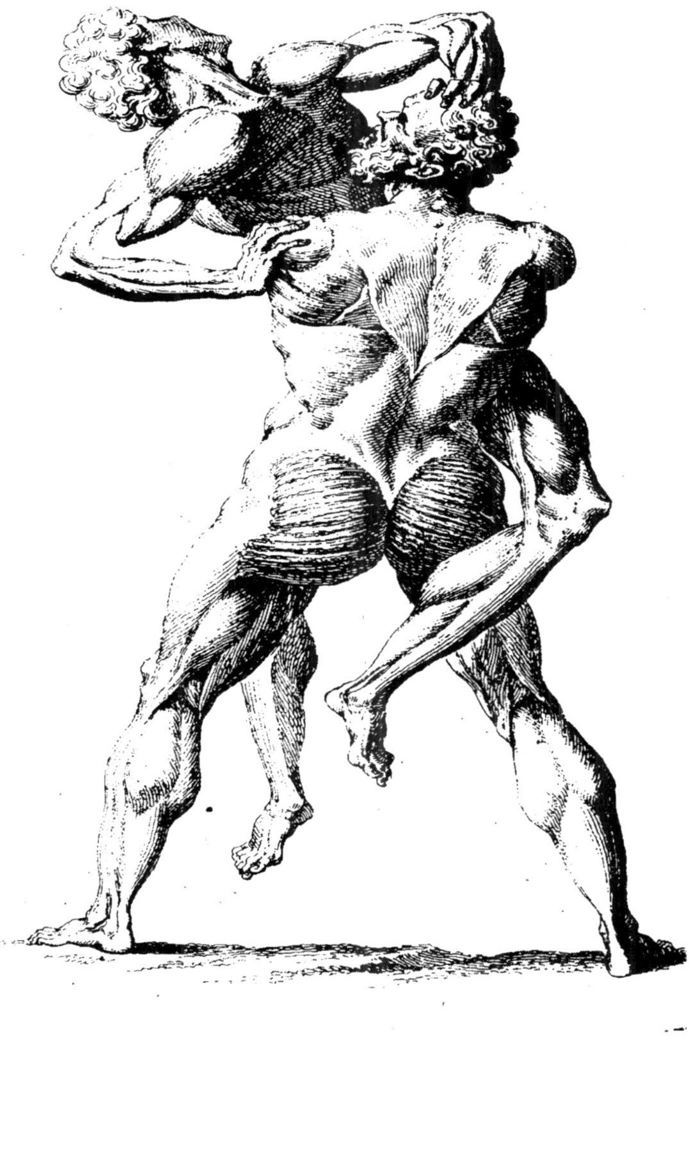

TAB. XX.

This table is done after the famous ſtatue of Hercules and Antæus. The muſcles here exhibited being all explained in the other plates, the figures are omitted to preſerve the beauty of the plate.

THE ANATOMY OF THE Human Body.

BOOK III.

CHAPTER I.

Of the external parts, and common integuments.

THE vulgar names of the external parts of the human body being ſufficiently known for the deſcription of any diſeaſe or operation; I ſhall only deſcribe thoſe which anatomiſts have given for the better underſtanding of the ſubcontained parts.

THE hollow on the middle of the thorax, under the breaſts is called ſcrobiculus cordis: the middle of the abdomen for about three fingers breadth above and below the navel, is called regio umbilicalis; the middle part above this, epigastrium; on each side of the epigastrium, under the cartilages of the lower ribs, hypochondrium; and from below the regio umbilicalis, down to the ossa ilia and ossa pubis, hypogastrium.

CUTICULA, OR SCARF SKIN, is that thin insensible membrane which is raised by blisters in living bodies. It is extended over every part of the true skin, unless where the nails are. It appears to me in a microscope a very fine smooth membrane, only unequal where the reticulum mucosum adheres to it, LEWENHOECK, and others, say it appears scaly, and compute that a grain of sand of the hundredth part of an inch diameter, will cover two hundred and fifty of these scales, and that each scale has about five hundred pores; so that a grain of sand will cover 125,000 pores thro' which we perspire. Its use is to defend the true skin that it may not be exposed to pain from whatever it touches; and also to preserve it from wearing: it is thickest on those parts of the bottom of the foot which sustain the body, and in hands much used to labour, being so contrived as to grow the thicker the more those parts are used. In scorbutic disorders the cuticula will sometimes become scurfy and full of little ulcers, which are apt to remain even when the cause is taken away, but the cuticle being taken off by a blister, the new cuticle will be found; and though the cutis is affected and

and full of little tumours, the discharge of the blister will often cure them also.

BETWEEN this and the true skin is a small quantity of slimy matter, which was supposed by MALPIGHI and others, to be contained in proper vessels, interwoven with one another, and therefore by them named reticulum mucosum. It is most considerable where the cuticula is thickest, and is black, white, or dusky, such as is the complexion; the colour of this and the cuticula being the only difference between Europeans and Africans or Indians, the fibres of the true skin being white in all men; but the florid colour of the cheeks is owing to the blood in the minute vessels of the skin, as that in the lips to the vessels in the muscular flesh; for the cuticula being made of excrementitious matter, has no blood vessels.

CUTIS, OF TRUE SKIN, is a very compact, strong, and sensible membrane, extended over all the other parts of the body, having nerves terminating so plentifully in all its superficies, for the sense of touching, that the finest pointed instrument can prick no where without touching some of them. These nerves are said by MALPIGHI and others, who have examined them carefully, to terminate in small pyramidal papillæ; nevertheless it seems that a plain superficies of the skin is much fitter and more agreeable to what we experience of this sensation; for a plain superficies exposing all the nerves alike, I think, would give a more equal

 sensation,

ſenſation, while nerves ending in a pyramidal papilla would be exceeding ſenſible at the vertex of that papilla; and thoſe at the ſides and round the baſe, which would be far the greateſt part, would be the leaſt uſeful. Immediately under the ſkin upon the ſhin bone, I have twice ſeen little tumors, leſs than a pea, round and exceeding hard, and ſo painful that both caſes were judged to be cancerous; they were cured by extirpating the tumor: but what was more extraordinary, was a tumor of this kind, under the ſkin of the buttock, ſmall as a pin's head, yet ſo painful that the leaſt touch was inſupportable, and the ſkin for half an inch round was emaciated; this too I extirpated, with ſo much of the ſkin as was emaciated, and ſome fat. The patient, who before the operation could not endure to ſet his leg to the ground, nor turn in his bed without exquiſite pain, grew immediately eaſy, walked to his bed without any complaint, and was ſoon cured.

GLANDULÆ MILIARES are ſmall bodies like millet ſeeds, ſeated immediately under the ſkin in the axillas; and are ſaid to have been found under all other parts of the ſkin, where they have been looked for with microſcopes. Theſe glands are ſuppoſed to ſeparate ſweat; which fluid was thought to be only the materia perſpirabilis flowing in a greater quantity, and condenſed, 'till SANCTORIUS aſſured us that it is not ſo, and that more of the materia perſpirabilis is ſeparated in equal times than of of ſweat; of the former, he ſays, uſually fifty two ounces a day in Italy, where his experiments were made, and of the latter not near ſo much in the moſt profuſe ſweats; which ſeems to favour the opinion of the exiſtence of theſe glands: but whoever reads Mr. HALES's experiments will find, that what SANCTORIUS accounted for by an imaginary inſenſible perſpiration, different from that which in the greateſt degree produces ſweat, is really made by the lungs in reſpiration, and is ten times more than all the ordinary perſpiration through the cutis, and ſeems to be but the ſame kind of fluid diſcharged both ways; for whenever it is interrupted through the ſkin in cold weather, then the lungs are overcharged, which occaſions coughing to get rid of it, which in a greater degree is an aſthma. Hence too it is that thoſe who perſpire moſt in the ſummer are moſt ſubject to aſthmatic diſorders in the winter: and moſt of all ſo, when the air they breathe is fulleſt of vapour, and therefore leaſt capable of conveying this matter from the lungs. That this kind of perſpiration is very great, is ſufficiently ſhewn by breathing upon glaſs, or any thing that is ſmooth and cold.

MEMBRANA ADIPOSA is all that membrane immediately under the ſkin, which contains the fat in cells; it is thickeſt on the abdomen and buttocks, and thinneſt neareſt the extremities; and where the muſcles adhere to the ſkin, and on the penis,

penis, little or none. It contributes to keep the inner parts warm, and by filling the interſtices of the muſcles, renders the ſurface of the body ſmooth and beautiful, and may ſerve to lubricate their ſurfaces. Whether the decreaſe of fat, which often follows labour or ſickneſs, proceeds from its being reaſſumed into the blood veſſels, or whether it is conſtantly perſpiring through the ſkin, and the leſſening of its quantity is from the want of a ſupply equal to its conſumption, is with me a matter of doubt, though the former opinion, I know, generally prevails. The cells of this membrane communicate throughout the whole body ſo much, that from any one part the whole may be filled with air. I have ſeen two caſes where the wind-pipe being cut, and the external wounds being cloſely ſtiched by injudicious ſurgeons, the air that eſcaped at the wound of the wind-pipe getting into the cells of the membrana adipoſa, blew up the upper part of the body like a bladder. The like accident I have ſeen from a broken rib, where, I ſuppoſe, the end of the rib had pricked the lungs; all theſe perſons died. In theſe cells the water is contained in an anaſarca, which from its weight, firſt fills the depending parts, as the air in the former caſes did the upper parts; and when theſe cells are very full, the water frequently paſſes from them into the abdomen, and after tapping, though the limbs were ever ſo full, they will almoſt empty themſelves in one night's

time.

time. This membrane is the uſual ſeat of impoſtumations and boyls, in both which nature, uninterrupted, always corrodes a hole in the ſkin; from whence we may learn, that the beſt way of opening any impoſtumation is by a hole, and that too as near the time of its breaking naturally as may be, that nature may make the utmoſt advantage of the diſcharge. There is ſometimes a large kind of boyle or carbuncle in this membrane, which firſt makes a large ſlough and a number of ſmall holes through the ſkin which in time mortifies and caſts off, but the longer the ſlough is ſuffered to remain, the more it diſcharges, and the more advantage to the patient; at the latter end of which caſe the matter has a bloody tincture, and a bilious ſmell, exactly like what comes from ulcers in the liver; and both theſe caſes are attended with ſweet urine, as in a diabetes.

MAMMÆ, the BREASTS, ſeem to be of the ſame ſtructure in both ſexes, but largeſt in women. Each breaſt is a conglomerate gland to ſeparate milk, with its excretory ducts; which are capable of very great diſtention, tending toward the nipple, which as they approach, they unite, and make but a few ducts at their exit. There are to be met with in authors inſtances atteſted of men giving ſuck, when they have been excited by a vehement deſire of doing it: and it is a common obſervation, that milk will flow out of the breaſts of new-born children, both male and female.

 THE

THE breaſts and uterus in women, the tongue, mouth, and penis in men, and the eyes in children, are the parts moſt ſubject to cancers; yet there is no part where this diſeaſe has not ſometimes fixed. It is a matter of diſpute among ſome ſurgeons, whether cancerous tumors ſhould ever be extirpated or not, though it is certain none of theſe ever were cured without, and being extirpated, there have been many. The objection againſt extirpation is this, that the operation often provokes the part, which otherwiſe might lie quiet: but I do not think this is true; in deſperate caſes, where we cannot extirpate, we find the beſt remedy is plentiful bleeding (which alſo is nature's laſt reſort) gentle conſtant evacuations by ſtool, and a vegetable diet; and though phyſic never cures while the tumor remains, yet after extirpation it is highly uſeful, and even the worſt conſtitutions have ſometimes been brought to their primitive ſtate. An eminent ſurgeon in the city, having a patient with a cancerated breaſt, extremely large, and ſo much ulcerated that the ſtench of it was inſupportable; ſhe inſiſted upon the extirpation, againſt all advice, with no other hopes but to be delivered from the offenſive ſmell. Sometime after the operation the wound looking extremely ſordid, he ſprinkled it all over with red mercury precipitate, which put the patient into a high ſalivation, upon which the breaſt grew clean and healed, the patient recovered, and, contrary to all expectation, lived many years

years in good health. From this accident I learnt the uſefulneſs of ſalivating, after extirpating cancerous tumors, though nothing is more hurtful before. In the extirpation of a breaſt, and all other tumors, as much ſkin as is poſſible ſhould be ſaved; for the loſs of a great deal of ſkin is ſufficient to make an incurable ulcer in the moſt healthful body, and much more ſo in a bad conſtitution.

CHAPTER II.

Of the membranes in general.

EVERY diſtinct part of the body is covered, and every cavity is lined with a ſingle membrane, whoſe thickneſs and ſtrength is as the bulk of the part it belongs to, and as the friction to which it is naturally expoſed.

THOSE membranes that contain diſtinct parts, keep the parts they contain together, and render their ſurfaces ſmooth, and leſs ſubject to be lacerated by the actions of the body; and thoſe which line cavitiesſerve to render the cavities ſmooth, and fit for the parts they contain to move againſt.

THE membranes of all the cavities that contain ſolid parts, are ſtudded with glands, or are provided with veſſels, which ſeparate a mucus, to make the parts contained move glibly againſt one another, and not grow together; and thoſe cavities which are expoſed to the air, as the noſe, ears, mouth, and

and trachea arteria, have their membranes beſet with glands which ſeparate matter to defend them from the outer air. Thoſe membranes that have proper names, and deſerve a particular deſcription, will be treated of in their proper places.

CHAPTER III.

Of the ſalivary-glands.

PAROTIS, OR MAXILLARIS SUPERIOR, is the largeſt of the ſalivary glands; it is ſituate behind the lower jaw, under the ear; its excretory duct paſſes over the upper part of the maſſeter muſcle, and enters the mouth through the buccinator. This gland has its ſaliva promoted by the motions of the lower jaw. Its duct paſſes over the tendinous part of the maſſeter muſcle, that it may not be compreſſed by that muſcle, which would obſtruct the ſaliva in it, though it is frequently ſaid that it paſſes over that muſcle that it may be compreſſed by it, to promote the ſaliva. In ſheep, horſes, &c. whoſe jaws are long, this muſcle is inſerted far from the center of motion, that the end of the jaw may be moved with ſufficient ſtrength, and that diſtant inſertion requiring a greater length of muſcle, that its motion may be quick enough, no part of this muſcle could be allowed to be tendinous; therefore, it ſeems, to avoid the inconvenience

nience of compreſſion from the muſcle, the duct in thoſe animals goes quite round the lower end of it. When this duct is divided by an external wound, the ſaliva will flow out on the cheek, unleſs a convenient perforation be made into the mouth, and then the external wound may be healed. I have ſeen patients with this gland ulcerated, from which there was a conſtant effuſion of ſaliva, till the greateſt part of the gland was conſumed with red mercury precipitate; and then they healed with little trouble. HILDANUS mentions the ſame caſe, which for two years had been under the care of a ſurgeon without ſucceſs; and was at laſt cured by the application of an actual cautery.

MAXILLARIS INFERIOR is ſituate between the lower jaw and the tendon of the digaſtric muſcle. Its duct paſſes under the muſculus mylohyoideus, and enters the mouth under the tongue, near the dentes inciſorii. I was at the opening of a woman who was ſuffocated by a tumor which begun in this gland, and extended itſelf from the ſternum to the parotid gland on one ſide in ſix weeks time, and in nine weeks killed her; it was a true ſcirrhus, and weighed twenty ſix ounces. In a man which I diſſected, I found a quantity of pus near this gland, and a bundle of matter not unlike hair, as large as an hen's egg.

SUBLINGUALIS is a ſmall gland ſituated under the tongue, between the jaw and the ceratogloſſus muſcle. In a calf I found ſeveral ducts of this gland

gland filled by an injection into the duct of the submaxillary gland; but MORGAGNI and others shew, that the ducts of this gland enter the mouth directly from the gland in several places near the grinding teeth.

TONSILLA is a globular gland, about the bigness of a hazel nut, situate upon the pterygoideus internus muscle, between the root of the tongue and the uvula. It has no duct continued from it, but empties all its small ducts into a sinus of its own, which sinus, when the gland is inflamed, may easily be mistaken for an ulcer. This gland with its fellow, direct the masticated aliment into the pharynx, and also serve for the uvula to shut down upon when we breathe through the nose. They are compressed by the tongue and the aliment, when the former raises the latter over its root, and thereby opportunely emit their saliva to lubricate the food for its easier descent through the pharynx. A scirrhous tumor of either of these glands is a common disease, and it admits of no remedy but extirpation. The best way of extirpating them, is, I think, by ligature: if the gland is small at its basis, the ligature may be tied round it, which I have often performed by fixing the ligature to the end of a probe bent, and so drew it round the gland, and tied it; and in a few days the glands dropped off; but meeting with other cases of this kind, where the basis of the gland was too large to tie, I contrived an instrument like a crooked needle

set

ſet in a handle, with an eye near the point; I thruſt this inſtrument, with a ligature into it through the bottom of the gland, and then taking hold of the ligature with a hook, I drew back the inſtrument; then drawing the double ligature forwards, I divided it, and tied one part above and the other below, in the ſame manner that I did to extirpate part of the omentum in the cure of an hernia, and this ſucceeded as well as the former: See the plate at the latter end of this book.

Pressure upon the ſurface of a gland very much promoting the ſecretion that is made in it, theſe glands are ſo ſeated as to be preſſed by the lower jaw, and its muſcles, which will be chiefly at the time when their fluid is wanted; and the force with which the jaw muſt be moved, being as the drineſs and hardneſs of the food maſticated, the ſecretion of the glands depending very much upon that force; it will alſo be in proportion to the drineſs and hardneſs of that food which is neceſſary; for all food, being to be reduced to a pulp, by being broke and mixed with ſaliva before it can be ſwallowed fit for digeſtion, the drier and harder foods needing more of this matter, will from this mechaniſm be ſupplied with more than moiſter foods in about that proportion in which they are drier and harder; and the drier foods needing more ſaliva than moiſter, is the reaſon why we can eat leſs and digeſt leſs of theſe than thoſe. What quantity of ſaliva theſe glands can ſeparate from the blood, in a given time, will be hard to determine, but in eating of dry bread it cannot be leſs than the weight of the bread; and many men, in a little time, can eat more dry bread than twice the ſize of all theſe glands; and ſome, that are not uſed to ſmoaking, can ſpit half a pint in the ſmoaking one pipe of tobacco; and ſome men in a ſalivation, have ſpit, for days or weeks together, a gallon in four and twenty hours; and yet, I believe, all theſe glands put together, do not weigh more than four ounces.

THE membrane which lines the mouth and palate, and covers the tongue, is every where beſet with ſmall glands, to afford ſaliva in all parts of the mouth to keep it moiſt; for thoſe more remote are chiefly concerned in time of maſtication. Theſe ſmall glands have names given them according to their reſpective ſituations, as buccales, labiales, linguales, fauciales, palatinæ, gingivarum, and uvulares.

A GLAND is chiefly compoſed of a convolution of one or more arteries of a conſiderable length, from whoſe ſides ariſe vaſt numbers of excretory ducts, as the lacteals ariſe from the guts, to receive in each gland their proper juices, as the lacteals do the chyle; and though the larger ſecretions are made by viſible glands, yet unconvolved arteries may alſo have excretory ducts for the ſame purpoſe. And this way, I imagine, ſecretions are made from all the membranes that line cavities, and ſome others.

There

There alſo ariſe from theſe arteries lymphatic veſſels, whoſe uſe ſeems to be to take off the thinneſt part of the blood, where a thick fluid is to be ſecreted, ſeeing they are found in greateſt plenty in ſuch glands as ſeparate the thickeſt fluids, as in the teſticles and liver; and it is obſervable, that where the thickeſt ſecretions are made, the velocity of the blood is the leaſt, as if it was contrived to give thoſe ſeemingly more tenacious parts more time to ſeparate from the blood. The arteries that compoſe different glands are convolved in different manners; but whether or no their different ſecretions depend at all upon that, I doubt, will be difficult to diſcover. The excretory ducts ariſe from the arteries, and unite in their progreſs, as the roots of trees do from the earth; and as different trees, plants, fruits, and even different minerals, in their growing, often derive their diſtinct, proper, nutricious juices from the ſame kind of earth; ſo the excretory ducts, in different glands, ſeparate from the ſame maſs of blood their different juices: But what theſe different ſecretions depend upon, whether the ſtructure of the parts, or different attractions, or what elſe, we have no certainty about, though this ſubject has employed ſeveral ingenious writers. For my own part, from the great ſimplicity and uniformity uſually ſeen in nature's works, I am moſt inclined to think different ſecretions ariſe from different attractions, ſeeing that in plants and minerals there ſeems to be no other way.

CHAPTER IV.

Of the peritonæum, omentum, ductus alimentalis, and mesentery.

PERITONÆUM is a membrane which lines the whole cavity of the abdomen. It contains the liver, spleen, omentum, stomach, guts, and mesentery, with all their vessels and glands; the upper part of it is no other than the proper membrane of the diaphragm, for there is no more reason to call that, part of the peritonæum, than there is for calling the membrane on the other side of the diaphragm, part of the pleura or mediastinum. The fore-part next the muscles of the abdomen, and their tendons, may be divided into two laminæ, yet, I think, anatomists in describing the duplicature or laminæ of the peritonæum have not always meant this division, but have taken the tendons of the transverse muscles for the outer lamina, and considered the other as one membrane, seeing that it is between these tendons and the peritonæum that the water is found in that kind of dropsy which is called the dropsy in the duplicature of the peritonæum. Upon the loins the inner surface only is smooth, and the outer part a sort of loose membrana adiposa, in which are contained the aorta, vena cava, vasa spermatica, and pancreas, with other parts of less note. The middle of the peritonæum upon the loins is joined to the mesentery in in ſuch a manner, as makes ſome account it a production of the peritonæum, and ſome part of the external membrane of the duodenum, becoming one membrane with the inner or ſmooth lamina of the peritonæum, and part of the rectum is covered in the ſame manner; but the kidneys and bladder of urine are contained in a diſtinct duplicature of this membrane. The dropſy of the peritonæum may be diſtinguiſhed by being leaſt prominent about the navel, for there the tendons and the peritonæum will not ſeparate; and the water in thoſe that I have diſſected, had made the parts where it was contained as foul as any ulcer; therefore none of them, I preſume, could have been cured by operation.

For the umbilical veſſels, ſee chap. Of the fœtus. For the proceſſus vaginalis, chap. Of the parts of generation in men.

Omentum, or cawl, is a fine membrane, larded with fat, ſomewhat like net-work: It is ſituated on the ſurface of the ſmall guts, and reſembles an apron tucked up; its outer or upper part, named ala ſuperior, is connected to the bottom of the ſtomach, the ſpleen, and part of the inteſtinum duodenum; and thence deſcending a little lower than the navel, is reflected and tied to the inteſtinum colon, the ſpleen, and part of the duodenum; this laſt part is called ala inferior; and the ſpace between the alæ is named burſa. This cavity is very diſtinct in moſt brutes, but ſeldom ſo in

 men.

men. Sometimes both alæ are tied to the liver, and, in diseased bodies, to the peritonæum. Its use is, to lubricate the guts, that they may the better perform their periſtaltic motion. MALPIGHI deſcribes adipoſe ducts in this membrane to carry the fat from the cells into the vena portæ, and thinks it a neceſſary ingredient in the bile. In dropſies of the abdomen, and in perſons who from any other cauſe have died tabid, it is generally rotten and decayed; and ſometimes the guts in theſe caſes adhere to one another: But whether theſe adheſions proceed from the omentum's ceaſing to perform its office, or from the periſtaltic motion of the guts being long diſcontinued through abſtinence, or both, I cannot determine.

DUCTUS ALIMENTALIS, is the œſophagus, ſtomach, and guts, viz. duodenum, jejunum, ileum, colon, cæcum or apendicula vermiformis, and rectum.

OESOPHAGUS, or gullet, is the beginning of the alimentary duct; its upper part is wide and open, ſpread behind the tongue to receive the maſticated aliment; it begins from the baſis of the ſcull, near the proceſſus pterygoides of the ſphenoidal bone, then deſcending becomes round, and is called vaginalis gulæ; it runs from the tongue cloſe to the ſpine, under the left ſubclavian blood veſſels, into and through the thorax on the left ſide, then piercing the diaphragm, it immediately enters the ſtomach. It is compoſed of a thin outer coat, which is no

more

more than a proper membrane to the middle or muſcular coat. The middle coat is compoſed of longitudinal and circular muſcular fibres, but chiefly circular, abundantly thicker than the ſame coat in the guts; becauſe this has no foreign power to aſſiſt it, as the guts have, and becauſe it is neceſſary the food ſhould make a ſhorter ſtay here than there. The inner coat is a pretty ſmooth membrane, beſet with many glands, which ſecrete a mucilaginous matter, to defend this membrane, and render the deſcent of the aliment eaſy.

VENTRICULUS, the ſtomach, is ſituated under the left ſide of the diaphragm, its left ſide touching the ſpleen, and its right is covered by the thin edge of the liver; its figure nearly reſembles the pouch of a bag-pipe, its left end being moſt capacious, the upper ſide concave, and the lower convex: it has two orifices, both on its upper part: the left through which the aliment paſſes into the ſtomach, is named cardia; and the right, through which it is conveyed out of the ſtomach into the duodenum, is named pylorus; where there is a circular valve which hinders a return of aliment out of the gut, but does not at all times hinder the gall from flowing into the ſtomach.

THE coats of the ſtomach are three; the external membranous, the middle muſcular, whoſe fibres are chiefly longitudinal and circular, the inner membranous, and beſet with glands, which ſeparate a mucus. This laſt coat is again divided

 by

by anatomiſts into a fourth, which they call villoſa. As the muſcular coat of the ſtomach contracts, the inner coat falls into folds, which increaſe as the ſtomach leſſens, and conſequently retard the aliment moſt when the ſtomach is neareſt being empty.

THE manner in which digeſtion is performed has been matter of great controverſy. The ancients generally ſuppoſed the food concocted by a fermentation in the ſtomach: But the moderns more generally attribute it to the muſcular force of the ſtomach; which Dr. PITCAIRNE has computed to be equal to a hundred and ſeventeen thouſand and eighty eight pounds weight; to which being added the abſolute force of the diaphragm and abdominal muſcles (but for what reaſon I am at a loſs to conceive, when ſo ſmall a part of that force can be exerted this way) the ſum then will be more than twice as much; a force indeed equal to the end for which he aſſigns it. Now this force of the muſcular coat of the ſtomach is near forty times greater than what BORELLI has aſſigned to the heart, which is much ſtronger; and Dr. KEIL has undertaken to prove, that the force which the heart exerts is not thrice as many ounces as BORELLI computes it to be thouſand pounds weight. Yet this is as certain, as that action and reaction are the ſame; that the abdominal muſcles and the diaphragm compreſs the ſtomach with no greater force than they do the liver and all other parts contained in the abdomen; and that the fœtus in utero, and all the

viſcera

viſcera in the abdomen, receive much more of this force, during the time of geſtation; and yet neither the fœtus, nor any other contained part, is digeſted by that force; and for the force with which the ſtomach itſelf acts, it will be juſt the ſame with the reaction of the food upon it, and therefore ſhould be as much more liable to be digeſted by this and the other force, than the food, as it oftner feels theſe forces than that (only that living bodies are not ſo liable to digeſtion as dead ones:) Beſides, it may be demonſtrated, that the force with which the ſtomach compreſſes any part of its contents, is not greater than what is given to equal parts of the contents in the ſmall guts; for if the moment of a muſcle is as its weight, and if the muſcular coat of the ſtomach does not bear a greater proportion to the muſcular coat of a ſmall gut, than their diameters bear; a ſection of the ſtomach having ſo many more equal parts to preſs than a like ſection of a gut, it will require juſt ſo much more force to give each part the ſame preſſure. Dr. DRAKE has ſuppoſed, that digeſtion is performed in the ſtomach, as in PAPIN's Digeſter; in which hypotheſis are contained all the abſurdities of that of PITCAIRNE, with this addition, that the ſtomach muſt be as irreſiſtible to diſtention at that time, as his iron pot, and the orifices as forcibly ſecured; but then indeed it ſhews how bits of bones, which dogs ſwallow, may be retained in the ſtomach without tearing it; which difficulty, in my opinion, Dr. PIT-

CAIRNE

CAIRNE has not ſufficiently accounted for, though it is none of the leaſt in his hypotheſis. In granivorous birds, where digeſtion is made by muſcular force, their ſecond ſtomach is plainly contrived for comminuting or digeſting their food that way; for beſides that it is one of the ſtrongeſt muſcles in their bodies, its inſide is defended with a hard and ſtrong membrane that it may not be torn; and theſe birds always eat with their grain the rougheſt and hardeſt little ſtones they can find, which are neceſſary for grinding their food, notwithſtanding it is firſt ſoaked in another ſtomach, and is alſo food of very eaſy digeſtion. In ſerpents, ſome birds, and ſeveral kinds of fiſh, which ſwallow whole animals, and retain them long in their ſtomachs, digeſtion ſeems to be performed by a menſtruum; for we frequently find in their ſtomachs animals ſo totally digeſted, before their form is deſtroyed, that their very bones are made ſoft. In horſes and oxen, digeſtion is but little more than extracting a tincture; for in their excrements, when voided, we ſee the texture of their food is not totally deſtroyed, though graſs, in particular, ſeems to be as eaſily divided as any food whatever, and the corn they eat is often voided entire: and in the excrements of men, are often ſeen the ſkins of fruits undigeſted, and ſmall fruits, ſuch as currants, unbroke, and worms alſo continue unhurt, both in the ſtomach and guts. Therefore, by comparing our ſtomachs with thoſe here mentioned, it appears to me, that our digeſtion is performed by a menſtruum, which is chiefly ſaliva, gently aſſiſted by the action of the ſtomach, and the abdominal muſcles, and by that principle of corruption which is in all dead bodies. For digeſtion is no other than corruption or putrefaction of our food; therefore meats preſerved from corruption by ſalt or ſpirits, are hard of digeſtion and unwholſome. Nevertheleſs, when this digeſting menſtruum of the ſtomach is too crude, the ſame ſalts or ſpirits, moderately uſed, become a remedy; and though meat long ſalted is ſo very unwholeſome, it ſeems not to be from the ſalt itſelf, but the meat made undigeſtible by being long ſalted; for thoſe who eat the greateſt quantity of ſalt at their meals are not ſubjected thereby to the ſame diſtempers. And this digeſting menſtruum, when the ſtomach is empty, exciting that uneaſineſs which we call hunger, our appetites and our digeſtion are thereby neceſſarily ſuited both as to time and quantity.

Duodenum is the firſt of the three ſmall guts; it begins from the pylorus of the ſtomach, and is thence reflected downward; it firſt paſſes by the gall-bladder, and then under the following gut and meſentery, and coming in ſight again in the left hypochondrium, it there commences jejunum, which is the ſecond of the ſmall guts; but the place where this ends and the other begins is not preciſely determined.

Jejunum

JEJUNUM is ſo called from its being found, for the moſt part, empty; it is ſituated in the regio umbilicalis, and makes ſomewhat more than a third part of the ſmall guts. It is diſtinguiſhed from the following gut by its coats, which are a ſmall matter thinner and leſs pale.

ILEUM is the continuation of the former, ſituated in the hypogaſtrium, and very often ſome part of it in the pelvis of the abdomen, upon the bladder of urine, eſpecially in women; it enters the colon on the right ſide, near the upper edge of the os ilium. This great length of the ſmall guts is evidently for the convenience of a greater number of lacteals, that the chyle which miſſes their orifices in one place may not eſcape them in another; but thoſe animals which ſwallow their food whole, and have it a long time in their ſtomach and guts, have ſhorter guts and fewer lacteals.

COLON is the firſt of the great guts; it begins at the upper edge of the right os ilium; thence aſcending paſſes under ſome part of the liver, and the bottom of the ſtomach, from the right hypochondrium to the left, and thence deſcends to the pelvis of the abdomen.

CÆCUM, OR APPENDICULA VERMIFORMIS, is ſituated on the beginning of the colon; it is leſs than an earth-worm, with a ſmall orifice opening into the colon: This gut has ſeldom any thing in it. In men it is called one of the large guts, though it is the ſmalleſt by far; but the miſtake ariſes

arises from copying the antients, whose descriptions of all the parts contained in the abdomen, seem to be taken from dogs; for in them, and in many other animals, it is very large: And some fish have them in great numbers, but very small; I have counted in a mackarell above one hundred and fifty.

RECTUM is the continuation of the colon thro' the pelvis to the anus. The lower end of this gut is the seat of the true fistula in ano, which usually runs betwixt the muscular coat and the inner coat; it is cured by opening it the whole length into the cavity of the gut; it is yet better, if it can be done, to extirpate all that is fistulous and scirrhous, for that is a sure way to make one operation perfect the cure. The other kind of fistula, improperly so called, is an abscess running round the outside of the sphincter, in the shape of an horse-shoe, being a circle all but where this muscle unites with those of the penis; this is best cured by opening and removing part of the outer skin. The first of these cases happens oftenest in full habits, proceeding frequently from the piles; the last is generally a critical discharge, and one of nature's last efforts in consumptive and scorbutic habits of body. The inversion and sliding down of this gut is called prolapsus ani, a disease common in children, especially those who are afflicted with the stone, and of not much consequence; in men it is more rare and more dangerous, being generally attended with a flux of humours. This case I have cured by taking away a piece a piece of the prolapſed gut with a cauſtic, length-ways of the gut; the wound diſcharged the flux of humours, upon which the gut was eaſily reduced, and cicatriſing in that ſtate it never more fell down.

I HAVE ſeen a caſe, where a bold unthinking ſurgeon, having cut off the prolapſed part, the cicatrix was ſo hard and contracted that the patient could never after go to ſtool without a clyſter, and then not without great miſery.

OFTENTIMES the piles occaſion large tumors at the lower end of this gut; theſe are always beſt extirpated by ligature; for if they are cut, they will ſometimes bleed exceſſively, and it is no eaſy matter to apply any thing to ſtop a flux of blood in that part.

THE guts have the ſame coats with the ſtomach; the fibres of their middle or muſcular coat are circular, or ſpiral, and longitudinal; of the latter, but very few. The antagoniſts to theſe muſcular fibres of the ſtomach and guts, are their contents preſſed from one place to another, and the muſcles of the abdomen, for theſe preſſing upon them alter their form into one leſs capacious; which neceſſarily extends their circular fibres. The great guts have three membranes, or ligaments, on the outſide, running their whole length, and ſupporting the ſacculi, into which thoſe guts are divided. The leſſer guts have, at very ſmall diſtances, ſemilunar valves placed oppoſite to the interſtices of each other, to prevent the aliment from paſſing too ſpeedily through the guts; and the better to anſwer that end, they are larger and more numerous near the ſtomach, where the food is thinner, than they are towards the colon, where the food is continually made thicker in its progreſs, by a diſcharge of part of the chyle. This contrivance, ſo neceſſary to men, becauſe of their erect poſture, when they are obliged, by ſickneſs or accidents, to lie along, becomes a great inconvenience, and calls for the help of clyſters and purges. But brutes have not theſe valves, becauſe they are not convenient in an horizontal poſture. At the entrance of the ileum into the colon, are two very large valves, which effectually hinder the regreſs of the fœces into the ileum. But clyſters have been frequently known to paſs them, and be vomited up; tho' the excrement that is ſometimes vomited up, I am inclined to think, is ſuch as had not paſſed into the great guts. The other valves in the colon are placed oppoſite, but not in the ſame plane, to each other, and make, with their anterior edges, an equilateral triangle; but as the gut approaches the anus, they become leſs remarkable, and fewer in number.

All the guts have in their inner membrane an almoſt infinite number of very ſmall glands: Theſe glands will, eſpecially ſome of them in the large guts, appear to the naked eye when they are diſeaſed: They are called glandulæ pyerianæ.

The length of the guts to that of the body is as five to one in a middle-ſized man; in taller men the

the proportion is uſually leſs, and in ſhort men greater.

Mesentery is a membrane beginning looſely upon the loins, and is thence produced to all the guts: it preſerves the jejunum and ileum from twiſting in their periſtaltic or vermicular motion, and confines the reſt to their places. It ſuſtains all the veſſels going to and from the guts, viz. arteries, veins, lymphæducts, lacteals, and nerves, and alſo contains many glands, called, from their ſituation, meſentericæ. The beginning of this membrane from the loins, is about three or four inches broad, but next the guts of the ſame length with the ſide of the guts they adhere to, which is in the ſmall guts about a fourth part ſhorter than the other ſide; but when this membrane is ſeparated from the ſmall guts, it ſhrinks, and meaſures about two thirds leſs.

I opened a boy, about twelve years old, that died of the iliac paſſion, vulgarly called the twiſting of the guts; the guts, ſtomach, duodenum, and jejunum were diſtended, with vapour and air, to near ten times their natural capacity, which ſo compreſſed the inteſtinum ileum, that nothing could paſs through it. The relations of this boy could give no other account of the cauſe of this diſeaſe, than that of his having eaten a large quantity of raw young carrots. This caſe happens very frequently to lambs that have been houſed, and turned out early in the ſpring to graſs, when the graſs is very rank and ſucculent; and alſo to horſes, oxen, and

and ſheep, when they happen to feed, by any accident, upon young beans or peas, or rich clover graſs, which are very apt to ferment in their ſtomachs. In theſe animals this caſe is commonly cured by running a knife into their guts; ſome inſtances of which I have ſeen, and have heard a great many reported; but this caſe happening very rarely to men, I believe that practice has never yet been uſed; though the inſtrument which is uſed for tapping in a dropſy of the abdomen, might do it with great eaſe and ſafety. Some anatomiſts, who have conſidered the impoſſibility of a twiſting of the guts, which is the vulgar name of this diſeaſe, have imagined that it proceeded from one gut being involved in another. Theſe involutions are found frequently in bodies that die a natural death, and without any inflammation, or any other ſymptom of pain.

CHAPTER. V.

Of the liver, gall-bladder, pancreas, and ſpleen.

THE liver is the largeſt gland in the body; of a duſky red colour. It is ſituated immediately under the diaphragm in the right hypochondrium; its exterior ſide is convex, and interior concave; backward towards the ribs it is thick, and thin on its fore-part, where it covers the upper ſide of the ſtomach, and ſome of the guts; the upper ſide of it adheres to the diaphragm, and is alſo tied to it and the ſternum by a thin ligament, which is deſcribed commonly as two; the upper part called ſuſpenſorium, and the anterior latum: but either of theſe names is ſufficient for it all. It is alſo tied to the navel by a round ligament called teres or umbilicale, which is the umbilical vein degenerated into a ligament; it is inſerted into the liver at a ſmall fiſſure in its lower edge. The ligamentum latum, or ſuſpenſorium, ſuſtains the liver in an erect poſture, or rather fixes it in its ſituation, while it is ſupported by the other viſcera, they being compreſſed by the abdominal muſcles; in lying down the teres prevents it from preſſing on the diaphragm; and in lying on the back, they both together ſuſpend it, that it may not compreſs and obſtruct the aſcending vena cava. It is nouriſhed by the branches of the celiac and meſenteric arteries in the liver, called arteriæ hepaticæ, but its blood veſſels, that compoſe it as a gland, are the branches of the vena portæ, which enters the liver, and diſtributes its blood like an artery, to have the bile ſecreted from it; and the branches of the cava in the liver, which return the redundant blood into the cava aſcendens: It has alſo ſeveral branches of nerves, and a great number of lymphatics; of which I ſhall treat in their reſpective places. Dogs and cats, and other animals, that have a great deal of motion in their backs, have their livers divided into many diſtinct lobules;

lobules; which by moving one againſt another, comply with thoſe motions, which elſe would break their livers to pieces.

THE gall-bladder is a receptacle of bile, ſeated in the hollow ſide of the liver; it is compoſed of one denſe coat ſomewhat muſcular, which is covered with a membrane like that of the liver; and is alſo lined with another, that cannot eaſily be ſeparated. Modern anatomiſts have deſcribed a number of ſmall ducts leading from the liver to the gall-bladder, by which they ſuppoſe the gall-bladder is filled; and theſe I thought I had ſeen in a human body that died of a jaundice, when I was a very young anatomiſt; but never being able to ſee any ſince in any animal, though I have made very diligent enquiry by experiments and diſſection, I am now perſuaded that there are no ſuch ducts; for if they are too little to be ſeen or filled by injections, I think they are too little for the end for which they are aſſigned. As to the argument for the exiſtence of ſuch ducts, which is fetched from the difficulty of the gall-bladder's being filled through the ductus cyſticus from the ductus hepaticus, I think it is of little weight, ſeeing the veſiculæ ſeminales are filled with a thicker fluid through a leſs direct paſſage. From the gall-bladder towards the duodenum runs a duct called cyſticus; and from the liver to this duct one called hepaticus, which carries off the gall this way, when the gall-bladder is full; then the ductus cyſticus and hepaticus being united,

 commence

commence ductus communis choledochus, which enters the duodenum obliquely about four inches below its beginning. The orifice of this duct in the gut is somewhat eminent, but has no caruncle, as is commonly said. As the liver, from its situation in the same cavity with the stomach, will be most pressed, and consequently separate most gall when the stomach is fullest, which is the time when it is most wanted; so the gall-bladder, being seated against the duodenum, it will have its fluid pressed out by the aliment passing through that gut, and consequently at a right time and in due proportion; because the greater that quantity of aliment is, the greater will be the compression; and so the contrary.

I KNOW no way of computing, with any exactness, the quantity of bile that is usually secreted by the liver in a given time; but if it is four times as much as all the salivary glands secrete, it may be twenty four ounces for every meal: to which being added six ounces of saliva, which, from what is observed in the chapter of the salivary glands, I think will appear a moderate computation: and supposing the pancreas in the same time secretes three ounces, there will then be thirty three ounces of fluids separated for the digestion of one meal; and that these necessary fluids may not be wasted in such quantities, they pass into the blood with the chyle, and may be soon separated again for the same use; and very likely, some of the same bile may be be employed more than once, for digeſting part of the ſame meal: And as the liver exceeds all the glands in the body in magnitude, and its excretory ducts ending in the duodenum, it ſeems to me to be much more capable of making thoſe large ſeparations from the blood, which are procured by cathartics, than the ſcarce viſible glands of the guts. The liver ordinarily weighs, in a middle-ſized man, about three pounds twelve ounces, the pancreas three ounces, and the ſpleen fourteen ounces. I have ſeen a diſeaſed liver in a man that weighed fourteen pounds four ounces; and in a boy but nine years old, that died hydropic, the liver full of hydatids, and cyſts of hydatids adhering to it, which together weighed ſeven pounds one ounce and a half, though ſeveral pints of water had been let out of it before. The ſpleen, in the ſame boy, together with the hydatids contained in its membrane, weighed three pounds. In a man I found a diſeaſed ſpleen, weighing five pounds two ounces; and in an old man, ſix foot high, I found a ſound liver weighing no more than twenty eight ounces, and the ſpleen but ten ounces: And in a man that had been cured of a dropſy I found a polypus very ſolid, almoſt filling the large branches of the porta in the liver, and a ſtone between the liver and gall-bladder, larger than a nutmug.

PANCREAS, the ſweet-bread, is a large gland of the ſalivary kind, lying a-croſs the upper and back part of the abdomen, near the duodenum; it

 has

has a ſhort excretory duct, about half as large as a crow quill, though it is commonly painted as large as the ductus communis choledochus: It always enters the duodenum together with the bile duct; but in dogs ſome diſtance from it; and, I think, always in two ducts diſtant from one another. The juice of this gland, together with the bile, helps to compleat the digeſtion of the aliment, and renders it fit to enter the lacteal veſſels. In a man that died of a jaundice, I found the ductus communis choledochus conſtricted by a ſcirrhous pancreas, the gall-bladder extended to the ſize of a gooſe egg, and all the ducts to twice their natural bigneſs. This is the caſe in which I thought I had ſo plainly ſeen the cyſtihepatic guts: I once ſaw the ductus cyſticus obſtructed, without the gall-bladder being diſtended, which, I think, furniſhes us with a very probable argument againſt the exiſtence of cyſtihepatic ducts. In thoſe who die of the jaundice, for the moſt part are found in the gall-bladder and the biliary ducts concretions of bile ſo light as to ſwim in water, yet are called gall-ſtones: Theſe cauſe the jaundice, by obſtructing the ducts; many of thoſe who have been cured of this diſeaſe, have had great numbers of theſe ſtones found in their excrements. A patient of mine, who had voided by ſtool ſeveral of theſe ſtones, had afterwards two of half an inch diameter, which made their way through the integuments of the abdomen, and was cured without much pain. Oxen, as the ſame gentleman informed

formed me, who have been long fed upon dry meat, abound with them; while others, fed with them, and afterwards turned to graſs, when killed, are found without them. This gentleman could never eat any herbs. He alſo informed me of a phyſician in France, that with great reputation cured the jaundice by giving his patients large quantities of the juice of herbs.

THE ſpleen is ſeated in the left hypochondrium, immediately under the diaphragm, and above the kidney, between the ſtomach and the ribs; it is ſupported by the ſub-contained parts, and fixed to its place by an adheſion to the peritonæum and diaphragm; it is alſo connected to the omentum, as has been obſerved. The figure of it is a ſort of depreſſed oval, near twice as long as broad, and almoſt twice as broad as thick. Sometimes it is divided into lobules, but for the moſt part has only one or two ſmall fiſſures on its edge, and ſometimes none; in its colour it reſembles caſt iron. The inner texture, in brutes, is veſicular, like the penis; in which veſicles are found grumous blood, and ſmall bodies like glands: But RUYSCH denies that the human ſpleen is of the ſame texture. The ſpleen I have ſeen taken out of a dog, without any remarkable inconvenience to him. I have twice, in a human body, ſeen three ſpleens, twice two, and once four; ſome of theſe were very ſmall, others nearly equal, but all together in any of theſe bodies were not larger than the one which is uſually found.

CHAPTER VI.

Of the vasa lactea.

VASA LACTEA are the venæ lacteæ, receptaculum chyli, and ductus thoracicus.

VENÆ LACTEÆ, &c. are a vast number of very fine pellucid tubes, beginning from the small guts, and proceeding thence through the mesentery; they frequently unite, and form fewer and larger vessels, which first pass through the mesenteric glands, and then into the receptaculum chyli. These vessels ere they arrive at the mesenteric glands, or in dogs the pancreas asellii, which is these glands collected, are called venæ lacteæ primi generis; and thence to their entrance into the receptaculum chyli, venæ lacteæ secundi generis. The office of these veins is to receive the fluid part of the digested aliment, which is called chyle, and convey it to the receptaculum chyli, that it may be thence carried through the ductus thoracicus into the blood vessels.

For the following excellent description, thus marked, " of the receptaculum chyli, and ductus thoracicus, I am obliged to Mr. MONRO.

" RECEPTACULUM CHYLI, PECQUETI, or
" SACCUS LACTEUS VAN HORNE, is a membra-
" nous somewhat pyriform bag, two thirds of an
" inch long, one third of an inch over in its largest
" part, when collapsed; situated on the first vertebra
" lumborum, to the right of the aorta, a little higher
" than

" than the arteria emulgens dextra, under the right " inferior muſcle of the diaphragm. It is formed " by the union of three tubes; one from under the " aorta, the ſecond from the interſtice of the aorta " and cava, the third from under the emulgents of " the right ſide. The ſaccus chyliferus at its ſupe- " rior part becoming gradually ſmaller, is contract- " ed into a ſlender membranous pipe of about a " line diameter, well known by the name of

" Ductus thoracicus. This paſſes betwixt " the appendices muſculoſæ diaphragmatis, on " the right of, and ſomewhat behind the aorta, " then lodged in the cellular ſubſtance under the " pleura; it mounts between this artery and vena " ſine pari, or azygos, as far as the fifth vertebra " thoracis, where it is hid by the azygos, as this " vein riſes forward to join the cava deſcendens; " after which the duct paſſes obliquely over to the " left ſide under the œſophagus, aorta deſcendens, " and great curvature of the aorta, until it reaches " the left carotid, ſtretching farther towards the " left internal jugular, by a circular turn, whoſe " convex part is uppermoſt; at the top of this arch " it ſplits into two for one half line, the ſuperior " branch receiving into it a large lymphatic from " the cervical glands. This lymphatic appears, by " blowing and injections, to have two valves; " when the two branches are united, the duct con- " tinues its courſe to the internal jugular, behind " which it deſcends, and immediately at the left

" ſide

" side of the insertion of this vein, enters the superior and posterior part of the left subclavian, whose internal membrane duplicated forms a semilunar externally convex valve that covers two thirds of the orifice of the duct. Immediately below this orifice a cervical vein from the musculi scaleni enters the subclavian. The thin coat and valves, commonly ten or twelve, of this duct, are so generally known, I need not mention them. In my notes I find little variation in the receptaculum, only its different capacities in different subjects, and sometimes more ducts concurring in the formation of it. The diameter of the duct varies in most bodies, and in the same subject is uniform, but frequently sudden enlargements or sacculi of it are observable. The divisions which authors mention of this duct within the thorax are very uncertain: In a woman I dissected last summer, at the eighth vertebra thoracis, one branch climbed over the aorta, and about the fifth vertebra slipped back again under that artery to the other branch, which continued in the ordinary course. Last winter I found this duct of a man discharging itself intirely into the right subclavian vein. The precise vertebra, where it begins to turn towards the left, is also uncertain. Frequently it does not split at its superior arch; in which case a large saccus is found near its aperture into the subclavian vein. Generally it has but one orifice, though I have seen two in one

" body,

"body, and three in another; nay, ſometimes it "divides into two under the curvature of the great "artery; one goes to the right, another to the left "ſubclavian; this however is very rare. The lym- "phatic, which enters the ſuperior arch, is often "ſent from the thyroide gland."

Supposing there ordinarily paſſes five pounds of chyle in a day through the lacteals, and that four ounces of this only are added to the blood (tho' it may be any other quantity for aught I know) and that a man neither decreaſes or encreaſes during this time, then all the ſeparations from the fluids and ſolids muſt be juſt five pounds; four ounces of which muſt be thoſe fluids and particles of ſolids, which are become unprofitable; and the remaining four pounds twelve ounces will ſerve as a vehicle to carry the four ounces off: So that we ſee for what reaſon more fluids are carried into the blood than are to be retained there, and how the body is by the ſame means both nouriſhed and preſerved in health.

CHAPTER

CHAPTER VII.

Of the pleura, mediaſtinum, lungs, pericardium, and heart.

PLEURA is a fine membrane which lines the whole cavity of the thorax, except on the diaphragm, which is covered with no other than its own proper membrane. The back part of it is extended over the great veſſels, like the peritonæum; and in regard this membrane paſſes partly under theſe veſſels, as the peritonæum does in the abdomen, they may be ſaid to lie in a duplicature of it; it ſerves to make the inſide of the thorax ſmooth and equal.

MEDIASTINUM divides the thorax lengthways, from the ſternum to the pericardium and pleura, which is a very ſhort ſpace, but in many brutes very conſiderable. It divides into two in men, but in brutes it is ſingle; it divides the thorax not exactly in the middle, but towards the left ſide, and is ſo diſpoſed, that the two cavities, into which it divides the thorax, do not end toward this membrane in an angle, but a ſegment of a circle; it hinders one lobe of the lungs from incommoding the other, as in lying on one ſide the uppermoſt might do; and prevents the diſorders of one lobe of the lungs from affecting the other.

THE lungs are compoſed of two lobes, one ſeated on each ſide of the mediaſtinum; each of which lobes

lobes are ſubdivided into two or three lobules, which are moſt diſtinctly divided in ſuch animals as have moſt motion in their backs, for the ſame end that the liver is in the ſame animals. They are each compoſed of very ſmall cells, which are the extremities of the aſpera arteria or bronchos. The figure of theſe cells is irregular; yet they are fitted to each other ſo as to have common ſides, and leave no void ſpace. Into theſe cells the blood-veſſels diſcharge a large quantity of lymph, or materia perſpirabilis, which at once keeps them from being dried by the air, and makes a large and neceſſary diſcharge from the blood, as has already been obſerved upon the ſubject of perſpiration through the ſkin. Dr. WILLIS has given a very particular deſcription of the inner texture of the lungs, but it is only imaginary and falſe, as he, and they who have copied his cuts and deſcriptions, could not but have known, if they had ever made the leaſt enquiry into the lungs of any animal; nor is his account of the lymphatics on the ſurface of the lungs, at all more true than that of their texture. In the membranes of theſe cells are diſtributed the branches of the pulmonary artery and vein. The known uſes of the air's entering the lungs, are to be inſtrumental in ſpeech, and to convey effluvia into the noſe, as it paſſes for the ſenſe of ſmelling; but the great uſe of it, by which life is preſerved, I think, we do not underſtand. By ſome the force of the air is thought to ſeparate the globuli of the blood that

have

have cohered in the ſlow circulation through the veins; and this opinion ſeems to be favoured by the many inſtances of polypuſes, which are large concretions of the globuli of the blood, found in the veins near the heart, and in the right auricle and ventricle of the heart; and their being ſo ſeldom found in the pulmonary veins, or in the left auricle or ventricle of the heart, or in any of the arteries; but if it is true that, while the blood paſſes thro' the lungs, many cohering globuli are ſeparated, yet it remains to be proved that theſe ſeparations are made by the force of the air. Dr. KEIL has computed the force of the air in the ſtrongeſt exſpirations againſt the ſides of all the veſicles, to be equal to fifty thouſand pound weight; which though we ſhould grant, we ſhall ſtill find the moment of the air in the lungs exceeding ſmall in any ſmall ſpace. For the velocity with which the air moves in the lungs is as much leſs than that with which it moves in the wind-pipe, as the ſquare of a ſection of the cells in the lungs is greater than the ſquare of a ſection of the wind-pipe; and therefore if the ſquare of all the extreme blood-veſſels in the lungs do not bear a greater proportion to the ſquare of the large pulmonary veſſels than the ſquare of the cells do to the wind-pipe, and if the blood in theſe large veſſels moves as faſt as the air in the wind-pipe, then the blood moving in the ſmalleſt veſſels of the lungs with a velocity equal to that of the air in the cells, the blood will have as much more attrition from

the

the power that moves it in its own veſſels, than the air can give upon them, as blood is heavier than air. Beſides, air preſſing equally to all ſides, and the globuli of the blood ſwimming in a fluid; this preſſure, be it what it will, I think, can be of little uſe to make ſuch ſeparations. Indeed it may be objected that the greateſt preſſure is in exſpiration, yet that ſurely cannot be very great, while the air has ſo free a paſſage out of them. Others have thought, that the air enters the blood-veſſels from the cells in the lungs, and mixes with the blood; but this opinion, however probable, wants ſufficient experiments to prove it; air being found in the blood, as it certainly is, is no proof of its entering this way, becauſe it may enter with the chyle: Nor is the impoſſibility which has been urged of its entering at the lungs without the blood being liable to come out the ſame way into the veſicles of the lungs, a good argument to the contrary; for if a pliable duct paſſes between the membranes of a veſſel, through a ſpace greater than the ſquare of its orifice, no fluid can return, becauſe the preſſure which ſhould force it back will be greater againſt the ſides of that duct than its orifice; which is the caſe of the bile-duct entering the duodenum, and the ureters entering the bladder. I think the moſt probable argument for the air's entering into the blood by the lungs, or rather ſome particular part of the air, may be fetched from a known experiment of each man in a diving bell wanting near a gallon of fresh air in a minute; and if pressure only was wanted in this case, they often descend, till the pressure of the air is three or four times what it is upon the surface of the earth, without any advantage from that pressure; and animals dying so soon in air that has been burnt, and their being so easily intoxicated by breathing air much impregnated with spirituous liquors, are also arguments of a passage this way into the blood. Besides, if pressure of the air in the cells of the lungs is the only use of it, I do not see but enough of that may be had while a man is hanging, if the muscles of the thorax do but act upon the air which was left in the thorax when the rope was first fixed, and yet death is brought about by hanging no other way than by interrupting of the breath, as I have found by certain experiments. Dr. DRAKE has endeavoured to shew, that the use of respiration is to assist the systole of the heart; but this use requires that the systole and diastole of the heart should keep time with exspiration and inspiration, which is contrary to experience. The lungs of animals, before they have been dilated with air, are specifically heavier than water; but upon inflation they become specifically lighter, and swim in water; which experiment may be made to discover whether a dead child was still born, or not; but if the child has breathed but a little, and the experiment is made long after, the lungs may be collapsed and grow heavier than water, as I have experimented, ed, which may ſometimes lead a man to give a wrong judgment in a court of judicature, but then it will be on the charitable ſide of the queſtion. Adheſions of the lungs to the pleura are in men ſo common, that I know not how to call it a diſeaſe; they being found ſo more or leſs in moſt adult perſons, and without any inconvenience, if the lungs are not rotten.

Pericardium, or heart-purse, is an exceeding ſtrong membrane which covers the heart; its ſide next the great veſſels is partly connected to them, and partly to the baſis of the heart, but, I think, not properly perforated by thoſe veſſels; and its lower ſide is inſeparable from the tendinous part of the diaphragm, but not ſo in brutes, in ſome of which there is a membranous bag between it and the diaphragm, which contains a lobule of the lungs. It encloſes all the heart to its baſis; its uſes are to keep the heart in its place, without interrupting its office, to keep it from having any friction with the lungs, and to contain a liquor to lubricate the ſurface of the heart, and abate its friction againſt the pericardium.

The heart is a muſcle of a conic figure, with two cavities or ventricles; its baſis is fixed by the veſſels going to and from it, upon the fourth and fifth vertebræ of the thorax; its apex, or point, is inclined downward and to the left ſide, where it is received in a cavity of the left lobe of the lungs, as may be obſerved, the lungs being extended with air. This incumbrance on the left lobe of the lungs, I imagine, is the cauſe of that ſide's being moſt ſubject to thoſe pains which are uſually called pleuritic, which I have ever found upon diſſecting of them to be inflammations in the lungs.

At the baſis of the heart, on each ſide, are ſituated the two auricles to receive the blood; the right from the two venæ cavæ, and the left from the pulmonary veins: In the right, at the meeting of the cavæ, is an eminence called tuberculum Loweri, which directs the blood into the auricle; immediately below this tubercle, in the ending of the cava aſcendens, is the veſtigium of the foramen ovale (vid. chap. Of the fœtus;) and near this, in the auricle, is the mouth of the coronary veins. Both auricles are ſtrengthened by muſcular columnæ, like the ventricles. The left is much leſs than the right; but the difference is ſupplied by a large muſcular cavity, which the veins from the lungs afford in that place. The ſides of this muſcular cavity are thicker than the ſides of the right auricle, in about that proportion, in which the left ventricle of the heart is ſtronger than the right; their uſes being to receive blood from the veins that lead to the heart, and preſs it into the ventricles, a ſtrength in each auricle proportionable to the ſtrength of the ventricle that it is to fill with blood, ſeems neceſſary: And this different thickneſs of the coats of the auricles makes the blood in the left, which is thickeſt, appear through it of a paler red; but when it is let out

out of the auricles, it appears alike from both; which they would do well to examine, who affirm the blood returns from the lungs of a more florid colour than it went in; and offer it as an argument of the blood's being mixed with air in the lungs. The ventricles or cavities in the heart which receive the blood, are hollow muſcles, or two cavities in one muſcle, whoſe fibres interſect one another, ſo as to make the preſſure of the heart upon the blood more equal and effectual, and are alſo leſs liable to be ſeparated than they would have been, if they had lain in one direction. Both theſe cavities receiving the ſame quantities of blood in the ſame times, and always acting together, muſt be equal in ſize, if they equally diſcharge what they contain at every ſyſtole, as I doubt not but they do; nevertheleſs the left appears leſs than the right, it being found empty in dead bodies, and the right uſually full of blood; which made the ancients think the veins and the right ventricle only were for the blood to move in, and that the left and the arteries contained only animal ſpirits. The left ventricle is much the thickeſt and ſtrongeſt, its office being to drive the blood through the whole body, while the right propels it through the lungs only. Over the entrance of the auricles in each ventricle, are placed valves to hinder a return of blood while the heart contracts. Thoſe in the right ventricle are named tricuſpides, thoſe in the left mitrales. One of theſe laſt ſeems to do further ſervice, by covering the mouth of the aorta while the ventricle fills; which ſuffering none of the blood to paſs out of this ventricle into the aorta before the ventricle acts, it will be able to give greater force to the blood than it otherwiſe might have done; becauſe a greater quantity of blood more fully diſtending the ventricle, and making the greater reſiſtance, it will be capable of receiving the greater impreſſed force from the ventricle; and if the blood is no way hindered in the right ventricle from getting into the pulmonary artery, while the ventricle dilates, as it is in the left, the left then may be ſomewhat bigger than the right, if they both empty themſelves alike in every ſyſtole. Though the auricles of the heart are equal to each other, and the two ventricles alſo equal, or nearly equal, yet the auricles are not ſo large as the ventricles; for the ventricles contain not only all the blood which flowed from the veins into the auricles, during the contraction of the heart, but alſo that which flows (which will be directly into the heart) while the auricles contract, and the ventricles dilate; which leads us to the exact knowledge of the uſe of the auricles. If the ſyſtole and diaſtole of the heart are performed in equal times, then the auricles muſt be half the ſize of the ventricles; or whatever proportion the ſpace of time of the ſyſtole of the heart bears to the ſpace in which the ſyſtole and diaſtole are both performed, that proportion will the cavities of the auricles bear to the cavities of the vintricles. The inner

fibres

fibres of each ventricle are diſpoſed into ſmall cords, which are called columnæ: From ſome of theſe ſtand ſmall portions of fleſh called papillæ; theſe papillæ are tied to the valves by ſlender fibres, whereby they keep the valves from being preſſed into the auricles by the action of the blood againſt them in the ſyſtole of the heart; and when that is over, the blood flowing in between them opens them, as the preſſure of blood on the other ſide ſhuts them in the ſyſtole. For the courſe of the blood through this part, vid. chap. Of the courſe of the aliment and fluids. In the beginning of each artery from the heart are placed three valves, which look forward, and cloſe together to hinder a regreſs of blood into the ventricles. Thoſe in the pulmonary artery are named ſigmoidales, thoſe in the aorta, ſemilunares. For the canalis arterioſus, vid. chap. Of the fœtus.

In a boy I found a great quantity of pus in the pericardium, and the baſis of the heart ulcerated. In perſons that have died of a dropſy, I have uſually obſerved the heart large, its fibres lax, and the veſſels about it immoderately diſtended, and polypuſes ſometimes in both auricles and ventricles, and in the large veins; but more frequently in the right auricle and ventricle. Mr. Pile has prepared a heart thus diſeaſed, whoſe circumference from the vertex round the baſe of the auricles meaſures twenty four inches and a quarter, and round the baſe of the ventricles ſeventeen inches and a half. I diſſected a man that died tabid, in whom the pericardium univerſally adhered to the heart, and a portion of the muſcular part of the heart was oſſified as large as a ſix-pence. The beginning of the aorta is frequently ſeen oſſified, eſpecially in aged perſons. In a woman that died of a dropſy, I found the valves of the aorta quite covered with chalk-ſtones, which not ſuffering the valves to do their office, the left ventricle of the heart was conſtantly overcharged with blood, and diſtended to above twice its natural bigneſs, which, I imagine, deſtroyed the œconomy of the body, and occaſioned the dropſy.

UPON opening the body of a perſon, who died with exceſſive palpitations of the heart and uneven pulſe, which began after very hard drinking, in extreme hot weather, ſome years before, I found about ten inches of the aorta neareſt the heart diſtended three times its natural diameter; and in a man one hundred and three years old, I found the ſame part of the aorta extended twice its natural capacity, without any ſymptom of ſuch a diſorder when living.

CHAPTER

CHAPTER VIII.

Of the arteries and veins.

FROM the right ventricle of the heart ariſes the pulmonary artery, which ſoon divides into two branches, one to each lobe of the lungs; then they ſubdivide into ſmaller and ſmaller branches, until they are diſtributed through every part of the lungs. From the extreme branches of the pulmonary artery ariſe the ſmall branches of the pulmonary veins; which, as they approach the left auricle of the heart, unite in ſuch a manner as the pulmonary artery divides going from the heart, only that the veins enter the muſcular appendix of the left auricle in ſeveral branches, and the blood being brought back from the lungs by theſe veſſels to the left auricle and ventricle of the heart, it is from the left ventricle of the heart thrown into the aorta.

AORTA, OR GREAT ARTERY, ariſes from the left ventricle of the heart, and deals out branches to every part of the body. The firſt part of this veſſel is called aorta aſcendens; it paſſes over the left pulmonary artery, and veins, and branch of the aſpera arteria, and being reflected under the left lobe of the lungs, it commences aorta deſcendens; which name it keeps through the thorax and abdomen, where it paſſes on the left ſide of the ſpine, till its diviſion

division into iliac arteries between the third and fourth vertebræ of the loins.

FROM under two of the ſemilunar valves of the aorta, which is ere it leaves the heart, ariſe two branches (ſometimes but one) which are beſtowed upon the heart, and are called coronariæ cordis. From the curved part of the aorta, which is about two or three inches above the heart, ariſe the ſubclavian and carotid arteries; the right ſubclavian and carotid in one trunk; but the left ſingle. By ſome authors theſe veſſels have been deſcribed in a different manner; but I believe their deſcriptions were, for want of human bodies, taken from brutes; for I have never yet ſeen any variety in theſe veſſels in human bodies, though I have in the veins nearer the heart: And indeed there ſeems to me to be a mechanical reaſon for their going off in the manner here deſcribed, in human bodies; for the right ſubclavian and carotid arteries neceſſarily going off from the aorta at a much larger angle than the left, the blood would move more freely into the left than the right, if the right did not go off in one trunk, which gives leſs friction to the blood than two branches equal in capacity to that one; ſo that the advantage the left have by going off from the aorta at much acuter angles than the right, is made up to the right by their going off at firſt in but one branch.

THE carotid arteries run on both ſides the larynx to the ſixth foramina of the ſcull, through which

which they enter to the brain; but as they pass through the neck, they detach branches to every part about them, which branches are called by the names of the parts they are bestowed upon; as, laryngeæ, thyroideæ, pharyngeæ, linguales, temporales, occipitales, faciales, &c. but just before they enter the sixth foramina of the scull, they each send a small branch through the fifth foramina to that part of the dura mater which contains the cerebrum. It is these arteries which make those impressions which are constantly observed on the inside of the ossa bregmatis: These branches, Mr. MONRO observes, oftner arise from the temporal arteries. The internal carotids send two branches to the back part of the nose, and several branches through the first and second foramina of the scull to the face and parts contained within the orbits of the eyes, and then piercing the dura mater, they each divide into two branches, one of which they send under the falx of the dura mater, between the two hemispheres of the brain, and the other between the anterior and posterior lobes. These branches take a great many turns, and divide into very small branches in the pia mater before they enter the brain, as if the pulse of larger arteries would make too violent an impression on so tender and delicate a part. And perhaps it may be from an increase of the impulse of the arteries in the brain, which strong liquors produce, that the nerves are so much interrupted in their uses throughout the whole

whole body, when a man is intoxicated with drinking; and may it not alſo be from a like cauſe that men are delirious in fevers? Beſides theſe two arteries, viz. the carotids, the brain has two more, called cervicales, which ariſe from the ſubclavian arteries, and aſcend to the head through the foramina, in the tranſverſe proceſſes of the cervical vertebræ, and into the ſcull through the tenth or great foramen. Theſe two arteries uniting ſoon after their entrance, they give off branches to the cerebellum, and then paſſing forward, divide and communicate with the carotids; and the carotid arteries communicating with each other, there is an entire communication between them all; and theſe communicant branches are ſo large that every one of theſe four great veſſels, with all their branches, may be eaſily filled with wax through any one of them.

The ſubclavian arteries are each continued to the cubit in one trunk, which is called axillaris as it paſſes the arm-pits, and humeralis as it paſſes by the inſide of the os humeri, between the muſcles that bend and extend the cubit. From the ſubclavians within the breaſt ariſe the arteriæ mammariæ, which run on the inſide of the ſternum, and lower than the cartilago enſiformis. Soon after the arteria humeralis has paſſed the joint of the cubit, it divides into two branches, called cubitalis ſuperior, and cubitalis inferior; which latter ſoon ſends off a branch, called cubitalis media, which is beſtowed ed upon the muſcles ſeated about the cubit. The cubitalis ſuperior paſſes near the radius, and round the root of the thumb, and gives one branch to the back of the hand, and two to the thumb, one to the firſt finger, and a branch to communicate with the cubitalis inferior. The cubitalis inferior paſſes near the ulna to the palm of the hand, where it takes a turn, and ſends one branch to the outſide of the little finger, another between that and the next finger, dividing to both, another in the ſame manner to the two middle fingers, and another to the two fore fingers. Theſe branches which are beſtowed on the fingers run one on each ſide of each finger internally to the top, where they have ſmall communications, and very often there is a branch of communication between the humeral and inferior cubital arteries. This communicant branch is ſometimes very large, and liable to be pricked by careleſs or injudicious blood-letters, in bleeding in the baſilic vein, immediately under which, as far as I have been able to obſerve, this branch always lies. Mr. MONRO has found the ſubclavian artery divided, in one ſubject, into two, the exterior of which formed the cubitalis ſuperior, and the inner artery, the cubitalis inferior; from which ſtructure he accounts for the ſucceſs in the operation of the aneuriſm ſometimes performed above the cubit. When the operation for an aneuriſm is made upon this communicant branch, it is found neceſſary to tie orifice, becaufe the blood is liable to flow freely into it either way.

From the defcending aorta on each fide is fent a branch under every rib, called intercoftalis, and about the fourth vertebra of the back it fends off two branches to the lungs, called bronchiales, which are fometimes both given off from the aorta, fometimes one of them from the intercoftal of the fourth rib on the right fide; and as the aorta paffes under the diaphragm, it fends two branches into the diaphragm, called arteriæ phrenicæ, which fometimes rife in one trunk from the aorta, and fometimes from the cœliaca; but oftener the right from the aorta, and the left from the cœliaca. Immediately below the diaphragm arifes the cœliac artery from the aorta; it foon divides into feveral branches, which are beftowed upon the liver, pancreas, fpleen, ftomach, omentum, and duodenum. Thefe branches are named from the parts they are beftowed on, except two that are beftowed upon the ftomach, which are called coronaria fuperior and inferior, and the branch beftowed upon the duodenum, which is named inteftinalis. At a very fmall diftance below the arteria cœliaca, from the aorta arifes the mefenterica fuperior, whofe branches are beftowed upon all the inteftinum jejunum and ilium, part of the colon, and fometimes one branch upon the liver. A little lower than the fuperior mefenteric artery arife the emulgents, which are the arteries of the kidneys: and a little lower than the emulgents, for-

ward

ward from the aorta, arise the arteriæ spermaticæ; for which, vid. chap. Of the parts of generation in men. Lower laterally the aorta sends branches to the loins, called lumbales; and one forward, to the lower part of the colon and the rectum, called mesenterica inferior. Between the arteria cœliaca, mesenterica superior and inferior, and the branches of each near the guts, there are large communicant branches to convey the blood from one to another, when they are either compressed by excrements, or from any other cause.

As soon as the aorta divides upon the loins, it sends off an artery into the pelvis upon the os sacrum, called arteria sacra; and the branches the aorta divides into are called iliacæ, which in about two inches space divide into external and internal. The iliacæ internæ first send off the umbilical arteries, which are dried up in adult bodies, except at their beginnings, which are kept open for the collateral branches on each side, one to the bladder, and one to the penis in men, and in women the uterus: the rest of these branches are bestowed upon the buttocks and upper parts of the thighs. The iliacæ externæ run over the ossa pubis into the thighs; and, as they pass out of the abdomen, they send off branches, called epigastricæ, to the fore-part of the integuments of the abdomen under the recti muscles: and the epigastric arteries send each a branch into the pelvis, and through the foramina of the ossa innominata to the muscles there-the iliac artery is paſſed out of the abdomen into the groin it is called inguinalis, and in the thigh cruralis, where it ſends a large branch to the back part of the thigh; but the great trunk is continued internally between the flexors and extenſors of the thigh, and paſſing through the inſertion of the triceps muſcle into the ham, it is there called poplitea; then below the joint it divides into two branches, one of which is called tibialis antica; it paſſes between the tibia and fibula to the fore part of the leg, and is beſtowed upon the great toe, and one branch to the next toe to the great one, and another between theſe toes, to communicate with the tibialis poſtica; which artery, ſoon after it is divided from the antica, ſends off the tibialis media, which is beſtowed upon the muſcles of the leg; the tibialis poſtica goes to the bottom of the foot and all the leſſer toes. The tibialis antica is diſpoſed like the cubitalis ſuperior; the poſtica like the cubitalis inferior; and the media in each have alſo like uſes. Theſe arteries, which I have deſcribed, are uniform in moſt bodies, but the leſſer branches are diſtributed like the branches of trees, in ſo different a manner in one body from another, that it is highly probable no two bodies are exactly alike, nor the two ſides in any one body.

I HAVE once ſeen a rupture of matter, and once of blood and matter, which flowed out of the abdomen into the fore part of the thigh, thro' the

the ſame paſſage at which the iliac artery goes out of the abdomen.

THE veins ariſe from the extremities of the arteries, and make up trunks which accompany the arteries in almoſt every part of the body, and have the ſame names in the ſeveral places which the arteries have, which they accompany. The veins of the brain unload themſelves into the ſinuſes (vid. chap. Of the dura and pia mater) and the ſinuſes into the internal jugulars and cervicals; and the internal jugulars and cervicals into the ſubclavians, which joining, make the cava deſcendens. The internal jugulars are ſeated by the carotid arteries, and receive the blood from all the parts which the carotids ſerve, except the hairy ſcalp and part of the neck, whoſe veins enter into the external jugulars, which run immediately under the muſculus quadratus genæ, often two on each ſide. The cervical veins deſcend two through the foramina in the tranſverſe proceſſes of the cervical vertebræ, and two through the great foramen of the ſpine, and one on each ſide the ſpinal marrow; theſe join at the loweſt vertebra of the neck, and then empty into the ſubclavians, and at the interſtices of all the vertebræ communicate with one another.

THE veins of the limbs are more than double the number of the arteries, there being one on each ſide each artery, even to the ſmalleſt branches that we can trace, beſides the veins which lie immediately under the ſkin. Thoſe which accompany the arteries,

arteries, have the ſame name with the arteries; thoſe which run immediately under the ſkin on the back of the hand, have no proper names; they run from thence to the bend of the elbow, where the uppermoſt is called cephalica, the next mediana, the next baſilica. Theſe all communicate near the joint of the elbow, and then ſend one branch which is more directly from the cephalica, and bears that name until it enters the ſubclavian vein; it paſſes immediately under the ſkin, in moſt bodies, between the flexors and extenſors of the cubit, on the upper ſide of the arm. The other branches joining and receiving thoſe which accompany the arteries of the cubit, they paſs with them by the artery of the arm into the ſubclavian vein. The external veins have frequent communications with the internal, and are always fulleſt when we uſe the moſt exerciſe; becauſe the blood being expanded by the heat which exerciſe produces, it requires the veſſels to be diſtended; and the inner veſſels being compreſſed by the actions of the muſcles, they cannot dilate enough; but theſe veſſels being ſeated on the outſides of the muſcles, are capable of being much dilated; and this ſeems to me to be the chief uſe of theſe external veſſels. The cephalic vein, as it runs up the arm, is very viſible in moſt men, but in children is rarely to be ſeen; therefore great care ſhould be taken not to wound it in the cutting of iſſues in childrens arms; and I know no way to be ſure of avoiding it, but by cutting the iſſue

iſſue more externally than is uſual in men; which may be done without any inconvenience.

In the thorax, beſides the two cavæ, there is a vein called azygos, or vena ſine pari; it is made up of the intercoſtal, phrenic, and bronchial veins, and enters the deſcending cava near the auricle, as if its uſe was to divert the deſcending blood from falling too directly upon the blood in the aſcending cava, and direct the blood of the deſcending cava into the auricle.

In the abdomen (beſides the cava aſcendens and the veins which are named like the arteries, viz. the emulgents from the kidneys, the lumbal and ſpermatic veins, the ſacra, iliac, and hypogaſtric veins) there is one large one called vena portæ, whoſe branches ariſe from all the branches of the cœliac and two meſenteric arteries, except thoſe branches of the cœliac and ſuperior meſenteric, which are beſtowed on the liver, and uniting in one trunk enters the liver, and is there again diſtributed like an artery, and has its blood collected and brought into the cava by the branches of the cava in the liver; this vein being made uſe of inſtead of an artery to carry blood to the liver, for the ſeparation of bile. It moves here about eight times ſlower than in the arteries hereabouts; and this ſlow circulation being ſuppoſed neceſſary, I think, there ſeems no other way ſo fit to procure it; for if an artery had been employed for this uſe, and been thus much dilated in ſo ſhort a paſſage, the blood would not have moved ſo uniformly in it, but faſter through its axis than near its ſides; and beſides, it is very probable that the blood in this vein, having been firſt employed in nouriſhing ſeveral parts, and having through a long ſpace moved ſlowly, may be made thereby fitter for the ſeparation of bile, than blood carried by an artery dilated to procure a circulation of the ſame velocity with that in this vein.

In the leg the veins accompany the arteries in the ſame manner as in the arm, the external veins of the foot being on the upper ſide, and from them is derived one called ſaphena, which is continued on the inſide of the limb its whole length, and has ſeveral names given it from the ſeveral places thro' which it paſſes.

The arteries have three coats; a middle muſcular, and an external and internal membranous. The veins are ſaid to have the ſame; the internal coat of an artery may be pretty eaſily ſeparated, but not the external; and though the veins have muſcular fibres, yet I could never ſeparate any one diſtinctly into three coats; and in the inſide of the veins there are many valves, eſpecially in the lower limbs, to hinder any reflux of the venal blood, which otherwiſe would have happened from the frequent actions of the muſcles on the outſides of the veins; and both the arteries and veins, as they run in the inſide of the limb, or as they are diſperſed in parts that ſuffer great extenſions, as the ſtomach, guts, and uterus, they are curved ſo much

much as that when these parts come to be distended, they may comply with those distensions by only being straightened, and so preserved from being stretched, which would lessen their diameters. The small arteries near the heart go off from the large trunks at obtuse angles, farther at less obtuse angles, then at right angles, farther still at acute angles, and near the extremities at very acute angles, because the blood in the vessels far from the heart moving with less velocity than the blood in the vessels near the heart, the blood in the collateral branches more remote from the heart wants the advantage of a directer course; and because a very large branch arising out of another, might weaken too much the sides of the vessel it would arise from, that inconvenience is prevented by increasing the number, and so lessening the size of the collateral branches, where otherwise one large branch would have served better; as in the going off of the subclavian and carotid arteries, which might have gone off for some space in one trunk; but this mechanism is more evident in the going off of the arteria cœliaca and mesenterica superior. And the small arteries always divide so as that the lesser branch may lie least in the direction of the blood flowing into them, which makes the blood flow most freely into that branch that hath farthest to carry it; and the smaller branches arise more or less obliquely from the sides of other arteries, according to the proportion they bear to the arteries they arise from, becauſe an artery comparatively large ariſing obliquely from the ſide of another, would make an orifice in that it ariſes from too large, and weaken it. And both theſe ends are at once brought about, by making the arteries, that give off the branches, bend more or leſs towards the branches they give off, according to the comparative magnitude of the branches given off.

Borelli has computed the force which the heart exerts at every ſyſtole, to be equal to three thouſand pounds weight, and the force which all the arteries exert at every ſyſtole, to be equal to ſixteen thouſand pounds weight, and that they together overcome a force equal to an hundred and thirty ſix thouſand pounds weight; and Dr. Keil has computed that the heart in every ſyſtole exerts a force not exceeding eight ounces. The firſt computation was made by comparing the heart with other muſcles, whoſe power to ſuſtain a weight could be beſt determined; and the latter was made from the velocity of the blood moving in an artery: Therefore if we conſider that Borelli's way of computing led him to find out the abſolute force of the heart, and Dr. Keil's the force which the heart uſually exerts, perhaps theſe very different computations may be accounted for; for if the force of the heart, which is conſtantly exerted, ſhould, compared with any other muſcle, be but in a reciprocal proportion to the frequency of their actions, and the importance of their uſes; may not the heart very

very fitly have a force vaſtly greater than uſually it exerts, becauſe it is always in action, and muſt be able to exert a certain force in the loweſt ſtate of health? What force the heart ever exerts in a grown man, I cannot ſay; but it muſt be leſs in each ventricle than is ſufficient to burſt the valves, which hinder the blood from returning into the auricles out of the ventricles, or than is ſufficient to break thoſe threads by which theſe valves are tied to the papillæ. In a dog, I found the force which the heart would exert, would not raiſe to one foot perpendicular height a column of blood through the aorta aſcendens. And when I inject the arteries of a child, I find a force exceeding little will throw water through all the veſſels, with a velocity equal to that with which the blood moves in thoſe veſſels when living. And if the heart, like other muſcles, can perform the firſt part of its contraction with moſt eaſe, are not the quick actions of the heart in hectic fevers owing to its not being able to empty the ventricles every ſyſtole, which, I think, will oblige it to act, cæteris paribus, ſo much the oftener? For the following ingenious attempt to account for the ſyſtole and diaſtole of the heart, and the reciprocal actions of the auricles and ventricles, I am obliged to Mr. Monro.

" Postulata, that the action of the muſcles
" depends on the influx of blood and liquidum
" nervoſum into the muſcular fibres, and therefore,

 " whenever

" whenever the muſcles are deprived of either or " both theſe fluids, their action ceaſes; this a great " many authors have fully proved by tying and " cutting the nerves or arteries that ſerve any muſ- " cle. That all muſcles are in a conſtant ſtate of " contraction as long as the blood and liquidum " nervoſum are freely ſupplied to them, which " ſeems evident from the ſphincter ani and veſicæ, " and from the continued contraction of ſuch muſ- " cles, whoſe antagoniſts are cut aſunder, or pa- " ralytic. That the nerves of the heart run to it " between the auricles and arteries, and that the " arteriæ coronariæ riſe from the aorta behind the " valvulæ ſemilunares, both which are evident from " diſſections. If then both auricles and ventricles " are ready, upon the firſt communication of mo- " tion, to contract at the ſame time, the ventricles, " as Dr. KEIL well obſerves, being ſtronger, will " firſt contract, and hinder the contraction of the " auricles, which muſt be in the mean time much " dilated by the influx of blood from the veins, " while the arteries are alſo diſtended by the blood " thrown out of the ventricles; therefore the car- " diac nerves lying between the two will be com- " preſſed, and the courſe of the liquids in them ſtop- " ped; at the ſame time the blood that ruſhes out " of the left ventricle into the aorta, puſhes the " valves of that artery upon the orifices of the ar- " teriæ coronariæ, ſo that no blood can enter into

" the

" the substance of the heart: Thus both causes of " contraction failing, this muscle must become pa- " ralytic. The resistance then to the contraction of " the auricles being now removed, they will throw " their blood into the ventricles; and the impulsion " of blood into the arteries from the heart now also " ceasing, the two great arteries will be constrict- " ed: The nerves are therefore now again free from " compression, and the valves of the aorta being " thrust back upon the mouth of the ventricle, the " blood enters the arteriæ coronariæ; since the ven- " tricles are again supplied with both the liquids, " on which their contraction depends, they must " again act. And thus as long as these causes con- " tinue, their effects must follow, i. e. as long as " the creature lives, the heart must have an alternate " systole and diastole, and the auricles and ventri- " cles have reciprocal actions."

If the arteries contract suppose a fourth part of the squares of their diameters at every systole, and if the heart does not throw out a quantity at every systole, equal to the fourth part of the solid contents of all the arteries when dilated, it is evident the heart does not throw the blood through the whole arterial system, but into so much of the arteries nearest the heart, as will contain four times as much as is thrown out of the left ventricle at once; and then this portion of arteries throws the blood forwards and dilates the arteries that lie next;

and ſo on: But if the capacities of all the arteries taken together in their utmoſt dilatations, exceed their capacities in their utmoſt contractions, juſt ſo much as the quantity of blood amounts to, which is thrown out of the left ventricle of the heart at every ſyſtole, which I believe is the caſe, then every contraction of the heart propels the blood through the whole arterial ſyſtem, which may be the reaſon why the largeſt animals, cæteris paribus, have the ſloweſt pulſes and leaſt vigour in their motions, and perhaps too for the ſame reaſon require a leſs proportion of food. The ſections of all the remoter veſſels being greater than a ſection of the aorta, the blood will move ſo much ſlower in the leſſer veſſels than in the greater, as the ſections of the leſſer veſſels taken together, exceed the ſection of the greater veſſel or veſſels. The ſtrength of the coats of the arteries, if the blood preſſed equally againſt the ſides of them all, cæteris paribus, ought to be one to another as their circumferences, becauſe ſo much as the circumference of one artery is greater than another, ſo much greater preſſure its ſides muſt ſuſtain; but the arteries neareſt the heart, ſuſtaining the re-action of all the arterial blood, they muſt have a ſtrength yet greater than in that proportion: And the veſſels, both arteries and veins, the more diſtant they are from the head, the greater proportional ſtrength their coats muſt have, becauſe the arterial and venal blood

commu-

communicating, they will preſs upon the lower veſſels, with a force proportional to the perpendicular altitude of blood above, which will be that of the perpendicular altitude of the whole body; for though the aſcending blood of the arteries may be ſaid not to preſs upon the deſcending, becauſe it moves another way, nevertheleſs it being thrown from the heart into one common veſſel, which afterwards divides, the blood moving both ways communicates, and that force which is neceſſary to overcome the natural inclination of the aſcending blood to deſcend, will be impreſſed alſo upon the deſcending blood, which is juſt the ſame with the weight of the aſcending blood; and the veins both from above and below communicating at the right auricle, the preſſure in them will alſo be as the perpendicular altitude of the body. So that the blood in all the veins and arteries may be compared to a fluid in a curved tube, in which that part in one leg exactly balances that in the other, and both preſſing moſt upon thoſe parts which are neareſt the centre of the earth. Accordingly we find by experience, that humours are moſt apt to flow to the loweſt parts, and that by laying thoſe parts upon a level with the whole body, this inconvenience is remedied; but laying a leg only on a chair does it but in part, juſt ſo much as the perpendicular altitude of the body from that part is ſhortened. There is alſo to be conſidered concerning the thickneſs of the coats of the veſſels, that the blood moving ſlower in the ſmall veſſels than in the great, the moment of the blood againſt the ſides of a ſmall veſſel will be as much leſs than the moment of the blood againſt equal parts of a great one, as the velocity of the blood in a ſmall veſſel is leſs than that in a great one; and therefore their coats may alſo differ from the former proportion, as the velocity of the blood differs. Moſt of the ſmall veſſels in the limbs lying againſt one another are a mutual ſupport, and therefore leſs liable to be dilated or burſt than capillaries which lie in the thin membranes of cavities, ſuch as in the noſe. Hence theſe, I ſuppoſe, are moſt ſubject to hæmorrhages. And if hæmorrhages of blood do frequently ariſe from obſtructions in the minuteſt veſſels, does it not appear how opium and the bark, if they thin the blood inwardly taken (as they do moſt powerfully when mixed with it) come to be ſo often effectual remedies in that caſe? And the coats of the leſſer veſſels being proportionably weaker than the great ones, according to the decreaſe of the velocity of the blood, which leſſens the moment with which it moves in them, whenever the blood begins to move in them with an equal velocity, or greater, as it happens after an amputation, when the larger veſſels are tied, the force of the blood ſometimes overcomes the ſtrength of the coats of the ſmaller veſſels, and dilates them ſo, that thoſe veſſels, which ſcarce bled during the operation, will ſometimes bleed afterwards. And this conſtant effort of the blood to dilate

dilate veſſels upon the obſtructions of others may cauſe thoſe throbbing pains which are felt in wounds when the bleeding is ſtopped, and in all violent inflammations, until the collateral branches are dilated, or the tenſion of the parts otherwiſe taken off.

THE extreme branches both of the arteries and veins have very numerous communications, like thoſe in the ſtamina of the leaves of plants, by which communications the blood that is obſtructed in any veſſels may paſs off by other veſſels that are not obſtructed; and the moment of the blood in the veſſels leſſening, and the friction from the veſſels increaſing as it approaches the extremities; and as many of the leſſer veſſels are more expoſed to preſſure than any of the large ones, thoſe communications in the leſſer veſſels are therefore made more numerous. By means of theſe communications, the blood circulates in a limb that has had part amputated, and into any veſſels that have been ſeparated from the trunks that ſupplied them, which otherwiſe muſt have mortified for want of nouriſhment, and with them, for the ſame reaſon, all the branches that ariſe from ſuch ſeparated veſſels; and I can diſcern no other way than by theſe communications, that the fluids contained in a large inflammation can ſuppurate into one cavity.

IF we inject by the arteries a large quantity of a coloured fluid, we find all the large veins full of that liquor before any of the ſolid parts are much coloured with it; and upon frequent repetitions all

of

of them much leſs coloured than, I think, might be expected, if it had gone into all the veſſels of the body; and I have often thrown wax or tallow, coloured with vermilion or verdigreaſe, through all the arteries, and back again through the veins, even to the heart, every where filling veſſels that cannot be diſcerned without a microſcope; and all this without filling or much diſcolouring any one entire part. In viewing with a microſcope the circulation of the blood in the tail of a fiſh, the eye eaſily traces arteries to their extremities, and their return in veins; yet all the veſſels we can ſee make but a ſmall part of the whole of what we ſee; though we are taught that the whole animal body is a compages of veſſels, ſuch as we ſee: But if it were ſo, I think, we could not well diſtinguiſh any; and if the ſum of the diameters of all the veſſels we can ſee, are to that of the breadths and thickneſſes of all the reſt of the parts, which we ſee at the ſame time, taken together, but as one to five, theſe veſſels then are no more than the twenty fifth part of what we ſee with them. What then ſhall we ſuppoſe the reſt of the tail, and thoſe parts which were ſo little tinged, and thoſe which were not filled with wax, in the foregoing experiments, compoſed of? Are they not compoſed of veſſels which ariſe from the arteries, as excretory ducts do in a gland, but terminate in the veins? And theſe veſſels being only to convey the nutritious juices, and what elſe may be a proper vehicle for them, is is it not fit the circulation in them ſhould be exceeding ſlow, that the nutritious particles may adhere the eaſier to the fibres of the veſſels, which they are to augment or repair? Beſides, if any whole part was made up of blood-veſſels, or any other veſſels with fluids moving ſwiftly in them, it ſeems to me impoſſible, that one part of a limb can be very cold while another part is hot, if the warmth of the parts is owing to the fluids they contain. And if there are ſuch veſſels as theſe, the velocity of the motion of their fluids will not depend upon any proportion they bear to the veſſels they ariſe from, but upon the velocity with which their fluids are ſeparated from the arteries into them, and the proportion of the ſections of all their orifices to the ſum of their own ſections, at any diſtance where we would compare the velocity of their fluids. And the ſtrength of the coats of theſe veſſels may not only be as much leſs than the ſtrength of the coats of an artery, as their diameters are leſs, but alſo leſs in that proportion in which the velocity of their fluids is leſs, and the motions more uniform, than the velocity and motion of the blood in an artery.

The coats of the veins are much thinner than thoſe of the arteries, comparing veſſels whoſe ſections are equal, becauſe the blood moving ſlower in the veins than in the arteries, it preſſes with leſs moment againſt their ſides: And beſides, the blood in the veins has nearly an equal uniform motion, but in the arteries a very unequal one; and that will

will require a farther difference in the ſtrength of their coats; for thoſe of the arteries muſt be equal to the greateſt natural preſſure; and if the arterial blood propels the venal, that is a farther reaſon for the different ſtrength of their coats.

All theſe things being conſidered, it appears to be a difficult thing to determine nearly, what proportion the fluids of an animal body bear to the ſolids, or what proportion the ſum of all the minuteſt arteries bear to the aorta, without which I think we can neither determine the comparative velocity of the blood moving in the different veſſels, nor the quantity of blood in any animal body, nor the time in which the whole maſs of blood, or a quantity equal to the whole maſs, is flowing thro' the heart. But if each ventricle of the heart holds five ounces of blood, and they are filled and emptied every ſyſtole and diaſtole, which I think is true, and if eighty pulſes in a minute be allowed to be a common number, there then flows twenty five pounds of blood through each ventricle of the heart in a minute. Dr. Keil has ſhewn that the ſum of all the fluids in a man exceed the ſum of all the ſolids, and yet the quantity of blood which all the viſible arteries of a man will contain, is leſs than four pounds; and if we may ſuppoſe all the viſible veins, including the vena portæ, hold four times as much, the whole then that the viſible veſſels can contain is not twenty pounds; but the whole that they do contain is but very little more than the

veins

veins can contain, ſeeing the arteries are always found almoſt empty in dead bodies. But how much the inviſible arteries and veins contain, I mean thoſe which contain ſuch a compound fluid as is found in the larger veſſels, I know no way to judge; unleſs we knew what proportion theſe veſſels bear to thoſe that carry the nutritious juices and ſerum (if there are ſuch) without the globuli of the blood. Cæteris paribus, is not the velocity of the blood in all animals proportionable to their quantity of action, and their neceſſity of food alſo in proportion to their quantity of action? If ſo, it appears how thoſe animals which uſe no exerciſe, and whoſe blood moves extremely ſlow in the winter, can ſubſiſt without any freſh ſupply of food; while others that uſe a little more exerciſe, require a little more food; and thoſe who uſe equal exerciſe winter and ſummer, require equal quantities of food at all times: the end of eating and drinking being to repair what exerciſe and the motion of the blood has deſtroyed or made uſeleſs. And is not the leſs velocity of the blood in ſome animals than in others, the reaſon why wounds and bruiſes in thoſe animals do not ſo ſoon deſtroy life, as they do in animals whoſe blood moves ſwifter?

I HAD a patient, whoſe muſcles on the inſide of the thigh were torn to pieces with the cramp, from whence was a vaſt effuſion of blood among the muſcles. The tumor being opened, it was judged neceſſary to take off the limb. The patient, a great diſcharge from the wound, was eaſy for about ten days; but the cramp then returned into the ſtump with ſuch exceſſive torment that he died ſoon after. I have never heard but of one other caſe of this kind, which ended in the ſame manner.

WHEN any of the veſſels are lacerated by bruiſes, ſtrains, or otherwiſe, without any external wound, purging (which is of more uſe than one can well account for) and cooling applications are always proper to prevent as much as may be extravaſations of blood or ſerum; but the lacerations once healed, which may be in eight or ten days, and the pain quite gone, then warm medicines may be applied, with opium, or ſp. cornu cervi (which powerfully ſeparate coagulated fluids) to help to attenuate and thereby diſſipate the extravaſated juices.

WHEN the blood-veſſels become unable to preſerve the circulation in the extreme parts, whether from particular weakneſs in the veſſels, or any other decay, I have always obſerved it to be hurtful to ſcarify. It lets out the juices that ſhould aſſiſt nature to make a ſeparation of the mortified part; nor can it be known in what place we may ſafely amputate till ſuch a ſeparation, which teaches us where it can be ſupported, and in any place ſhort of that an operation will be both uſeleſs and miſchievous. I have known many ſucceed well who have been thus left to ſeparate, but very few that were otherwiſe treated; nay, have known ſome

extra-

extraordinary inſtances of ſucceſs where the patient had the happineſs to have no one about them to interrupt the kind aſſiſtance of nature.

CHAPTER X.

Of the lymphæducts.

LYMPHÆDUCTS are ſmall pellucid cylindrical tubes, which ariſe inviſible from the extremities of the arteries throughout the whole body, but more plentifully in glands than other parts, and in greateſt number from ſuch glands as ſeparate the moſt viſcid fluids, as may be obſerved in the liver and teſtes. They cannot be diſcerned in a natural ſtate to have more than one coat, and that exceeding thin, having valves at ſmall and uncertain diſtances, to prevent the regreſs of their fluid. They have frequent communications like the veins, but do not unite ſo often; the larger trunks are in many places attended with ſmall glands, thro' which they run, and at the ſame time ſend communicant branches over them, that they might be ſecured againſt obſtructions from diſeaſes in thoſe glands. They all terminate in the vaſa lactea, or in the large veins. All that riſe in the abdomen empty into the venæ lacteæ ſecundi generis and receptaculum chyli; thoſe in the cavity of the thorax into the ductus thoracicus and the ſubclavian veins. Their uſes are to carry lymph to dilute the chyle, to make it incorporate more readily with the blood (but not to make it flow the better in the lacteals, as appears sufficiently from their not entering into the minutest lacteals) and to carry off so much lymph as is necessary to leave the blood in fit temper to flow through the veins; for it is always observed that in such persons as have their blood too thin, the globuli cohere and form moleculæ, or polypuses, which I imagine may arise from the globuli of the blood not rubbing often enough, and with sufficient force one against another to disunite them as fast as they cohere. These polypuses are frequently found in all the large veins, and in the right auricle and ventricle of the heart, especially in such bodies as die hydropic or of any chronic diseases.

Authors have described and painted these vessels as they appear when injected with mercury; in which case the coat of these vessels being exceeding thin, it is not able any where between the valves to resist the mercury's attracting itself into globules: And the same appearance also happens when they are vastly distended; because the valves hindering a distension where they are seated, the spaces between them approach to a spherical figure from the equal pressure of the fluid, according to the degree of their distension: but in a natural state, when they are filled with lymph, or when they are moderately injected with air or water, they appear as cylindrical as the veins. Any of these vessels being burst,

burſt, they cauſe a dropſy in the cavity into which they open, which is oftner in the abdomen than the thorax. This kind of dropſy is ſometimes cured by tapping; and I believe the reaſon why it no oftner ſucceeds is, that it generally takes its riſe from a diſeaſed liver. Formerly in this operation only part of the water was drawn off at a time, and the tap ſometimes left in the wound to draw off more, which was exceeding painful, and ſometimes brought on a mortification; and if they drew off much water at one time the patient was in great pain, and generally fainted, which was thought to proceed from the loſs of too much of the liquor at once. But Dr. MEAD, obſerving that theſe ſymptoms could not proceed from the loſs of an extravaſated fluid, ſoon found the true cauſe, which was the ſudden want of the preſſure of the abdominal muſcles againſt the parts contained in the abdomen; and in the year 1705, being then phyſician to St. Thomas's hoſpital, ordered it to be tried there in the following manner: He directed the abdomen to be preſſed by the hands of aſſiſtants while the water was running out, and afterwards kept rolled till the muſcles recovered force to do their office, and ſo took out all the water at once without any inconvenience, which has made this operation not very painful, ſometimes ſucceſsful, and never dangerous. I preſerved one woman, by ſixteen operations, from the fifty ſixth year of her age to eighty; another ſix years by ſixty ſix tappings: It must be confessed, that few cases suceeed like these, and very few recover.

I OPENED a woman, who died of a dropsy in the liver, in which I found the gibbous part entirely wasted, and the coat of the liver about a quarter of an inch thick, which contained about five gallons of a gross yellowish fluid, in which were many hydatids about the size of gooseberries, and some pieces of matter of as bright a red as vermilion. At about fourteen years of age she first began to feel pain in this part, which returned monthly, but in time grew continual, her belly constantly increasing till she died, which was in the twenty-eight year of her age, without ever having had her menses. All the other viscera both in the thorax and abdomen were perfectly sound, nor was there the least sign of the dropsy in any of the limbs, or yellowness in the skin, which is frequent in diseases of the liver.

CHAPTER XI.

Of the lymphatic glands.

THE glands accompanying the lymphatics are situated in the three cavities, in the interstices of the muscles, where the lymphatics lie with the large blood-vessels, and in the four emunctories, viz. the arm-pits and groins. In the brain is is ſeated the glandula pinealis, which I judge to be of this ſort, having often ſeen large lymphæducts running into it from the plexus choroides; and at the baſis of the brain in the cella turcica is the glandula pituitaria, into which enters a large lymphatic, as I imagine, named infundibulum (vid. chap. Of the brain.) In the neck are ſituated a great many of theſe, by the ſides of the carotid arteries and internal jugular veins, and two, or a ſort of double one, upon the larynx, immediately below the thyroid cartilage, from which ſituation they derive the name of thyroideæ; and juſt within the thorax is ſeated another, called thymus. In very young children the thymus is as large, or larger, than the thyroid glands; but in men theſe glands are very large, and the thymus very ſmall, the former having increaſed in about a double proportion of any other gland of this kind, and the latter having rather diminiſhed than increaſed: But in brutes, ſuch as have fallen under my obſervation, it is juſt the contrary. From which obſervations I am inclined to conclude, that they both belong to the very ſame lymphatics, and that either of them increaſing as much as both ought to do if both increaſed, anſwers the ſame end as if both did; and that the reaſon why the thymus increaſes rather than the thyroid glands in brutes, is becauſe the ſhape of their thorax affords convenient room for it to lodge in; and that in men the thyroid glands increaſed ſo much, becauſe there is no room in that part of the

the thorax where the thymus is ſeated for a large gland to be lodged. In dogs, a porpoiſe, and ſome other animals, I have ſeen the lymphatics in the thymus, and between the thymus and ductus thoracicus, full of chyle, and ſo in many other lymphatics near the vaſa lactea. Under the baſis of the heart, and at the ſides of the lungs, where the great veſſels enter, are many of theſe glands, from the ſize of a pea to that of a hazel nut. In the abdomen, upon the loins, near the kidneys, and by the ſides of the iliac veſſels, are many of theſe glands, which are called lumbales; and there are ſome at the hollow ſide of the liver, named hepaticæ: The meſentery alſo is full of glands of a like appearance, but theſe ſeem to belong only to the lacteal veins, unleſs ſome of them, which are ſeated at the baſis of the meſentery, among the venæ lacteæ ſecundi generis, belong to the lymphatics that come from the liver, where the hepatic lymphatics paſs in their way to the receptaculum chyli. The glands which accompany the blood-veſſels in the limbs are few, and diſtributed in no certain order; except thoſe in the four emunctories, i. e. in the arm-pits and groins, named axillares and inguinales.

Brutes have one large one in the thigh, commonly called the pope's-eye; this is ſeated about the great veſſels in the thigh, where they paſs through the triceps muſcle. From this ſituation, and not from any thing extraordinary in this gland, it is that wounds are there ſo dangerous.

The

The lymphatic glands are ſaid by NUCK, and others after him, to be compoſed of veſicles, and not of veſſels like other glands; and that theſe veſicles are repoſitories of lymph: But from their appearance in a natural ſtate, which is very compact and uniform, there ſeems to me to be but little reaſon for ſuch a conjecture. Some have thought their uſe to be by contracting to accelerate the motion of the fluid in the lymphatics; but that does not ſeem very probable, becauſe a muſcular coat would have been the readieſt means to produce that effect; beſides, theſe veſſels ſeldom enter any of them without detaching a branch over at the ſame time, perhaps to prevent obſtructions. And if theſe glands were endued with a contracting power, which is only preſumed without any proof, it would ſtill be difficult to conceive how ſuch a power, applied at uncertain ſpaces, ſhould not rather obſtruct than accelerate the motion of lymph in the lymphatics, unleſs there were valves to prevent a reflux; and even then, if this were a convenient piece of mechaniſm, it would be ſtrange it ſhould no where elſe in the body be made uſe of.

THESE lymphatic glands being diſeaſed, are apt to obſtruct and occaſion the burſting of the lymphatics that paſs through them; which, if in the breaſt, cauſes an incurable hydrops pectoris; if in the abdomen, the true aſcites, attended with a waſting of the limbs, which is never cured, but may be relieved by tapping.

CHAP. XII.

Of the course of the aliment and fluids, abstracted from the foregoing chapters.

THE aliment being received into the mouth, is there masticated, and impregnated with saliva, which is pressed out of the salivary glands by the motions of the jaw and the muscles that move it and the tongue. Then it descends through the pharynx into the stomach, where it is digested by the juices of the stomach (which are what is thrown out of the glands of its inmost coat, and saliva out of the mouth) and a moderate warmth and attrition. Then it is thrown through the pylorus or right orifice of the stomach into the duodenum, where it is mixed with bile from the gall-bladder and liver, and the pancreatic juice from the pancreatic gland. These fluids serve farther to attenuate and dilute the digested aliment, and probably, to make the fluid part separate better from the fæces. After this it is continually moved by the peristaltic motion of the guts, and the compression of the diaphragm and abdominal muscles, by which forces the fluid parts are pressed into the lacteals, and the gross parts through the guts to the anus.

THE chyle, or thin and milky part of the aliment, being received into the lacteals from all the ſmall guts, they carry it into the receptaculum chyli, and from thence the ductus thoracicus carries it into the left ſubclavian vein, where it mixes with the blood, and paſſes with it to the heart.

All the veins being emptied into two branches, viz. the aſcending and deſcending cava, they empty into the right auricle of the heart; the right auricle unloads into the right ventricle, which throws the blood through the pulmonary artery into the lungs; from the lungs the blood is brought by the pulmonary veins into the left auricle, and from that into the left ventricle, by which it is thrown into the aorta, and diſtributed through the body. From the extremities of the arteries ariſe the veins and lymphatics; the veins to collect the blood and bring it back to the heart; and the lymphatics to return the lymph, or thinner part of the blood, from the arteries to the veins and the vaſa lactea, where it mixes with the chyle, and then paſſes with it into the left ſubclavian vein and to the heart.

All the fluids that paſs into the ſtomach and guts being carried into the blood-veſſels, the greateſt part of them are ſeparated and carried off by proper veſſels, viz. urine from the kidneys, bile from the liver, &c. and theſe juices carry along with them whatever might be injurious to the animal œconomy.

CHAPTER

CHAPTER XIII.

Of the dura mater and pia mater.

DURA MATER is a very compact ſtrong membrane, lining the inſide of the ſcull, firmly adhering at its baſis, and but lightly at the upper part, except at the ſutures. It has three proceſſes; the firſt, named falx, begins at the criſta galli, and runs backwards under the ſutura ſagittalis to the cerebellum, dividing the cerebrum into two hemiſpheres. Its uſe is ſaid to be to ſupport one ſide of the cerebrum from preſſing on the other when the head is inclined to one ſide. But I think it is evident that this is not the uſe, becauſe there would be more need of ſuch a proceſs from one ſide of the ſcull to the other, than this way; and it would alſo be very neceſſary that it ſhould run through the brain, to anſwer that end. The principal uſe appears to me to be, to divide the brain into ſuch portions as are leaſt liable to be moved in the ſcull, by any violent motions of the head, which is better done this way than it would the other; and the under-ſide of the brain is kept ſteddy by the inequalities of the baſis of the ſcull, which the brain is exactly fitted to. In brutes the falx is always very ſmall, therefore in thoſe whoſe brains are of the larger ſize, as oxen, ſheep, horſes, &c. the upper part of the ſcull is made uneven, exactly to fit the folds of the brain, which ſecures the

the upper parts of their brains from concuſſions, in the ſame manner that the lower parts are ſecured. The ſecond proceſs runs from the lower and back part of the former to the upper edge of each os petroſum, and ſuſtains the poſterior lobes of the cerebrum, that they might not compreſs the cerebellum. In ſuch rapacious animals as I have diſſected, this proceſs is bone. The third is very ſmall; it runs from the laſt deſcribed proceſs down towards the great foramen of the ſcull, and poſſeſſes the ſmall ſpace in the cerebellum, between the proceſſus vermiformis. Theſe proceſſes of the dura mater alſo ſerve to keep the brain ſteddy.

THE dura mater has in it ſeveral ſinuſes, which are large veins to receive the blood from the leſſer veins of the brain: Their number is uncertain, and thoſe that are conſtant are not deſcribed in the ſame order by writers. The firſt that preſents itſelf is the longitudinalis ſuperior, running from a blind hole a little above the criſta galli all along the upper edge of the falx. A tranſverſe ſection of this veſſel is not circular, like other veſſels, but a triangle, whoſe ſides are arches of a circle; the upper ſide convex outwards, and the two lower convex inwards. The figure of this veſſel is preſerved by ſmall ligaments running acroſs in the inſide, that it might not become conical, or cylindrical, like other veſſels, from the equal preſſure of the contained blood, and thereby incommode the

upper

upper edges of each hemiſphere of the cerebrum. On the lower edge of this proceſs is generally another very ſmall one, called longitudinalis inferior; this runs into the rectus, and when wanting is ſupplied by a vein; the rectus runs between the two firſt proceſſes of the dura mater, and unloads with the ſinus longitudinalis ſuperior into the two lateral ſinuſes; but for the moſt part the longitudinal ſinus goes more directly into one of the lateral ſinuſes, and the ſtrait ſinus into the other. There is ſometimes a ſmall one in the third proceſs, which empties in the ſame place with the former. From the endings of the longitudinal and ſtrait ſinuſes, begin the two lateral ſinuſes, which, when they come to the os petroſum, dip down and paſs thro' the eighth foramina into the internal jugular veins. There is another named circularis; it runs round the fore part only of the ſella turcica; the two ends of this empty into four ſinuſes, one on the top of each os petroſum, which paſs into the ſinus laterales, and one at the under ſides of the ſame bones, which paſs indifferently into both the lateral and cervical ſinuſes; theſe two laſt ſinuſes have always communicant branches. The cervical ſinuſes run from the baſis of the ſcull through the great foramen on both ſides of the medulla ſpinalis colli, and through the tranſverſe proceſſes of the cervical vertebræ; the laſt of theſe have many times proper foramina running from the eighth foramina

to

to the back part of the apophyſes of the occipital bone. There are alſo two more of theſe veſſels, which run from the circular ſinus between the os ſphenoides and fore part of the os petroſum directly into the internal jugular veins.

PIA MATER is an exceeding fine membrane immediately inveſting the brain, even between its lobes, hemiſpheres, and folds. It ſerves to contain the brain, and ſupport its blood-veſſels, which run here in great numbers, for the arteries to divide into ſmall branches upon, that the blood may not enter the brain too impetuouſly; and for the veins to unite on, that they may enter the ſinuſes in fewer and larger branches. Between the dura and pia mater, is deſcribed, by ſeveral anatomiſts, a membrane called arachnoides, which may eaſily be ſhewn at the back part of the cerebrum, upon the cerebellum and back part of the medulla ſpinalis.

I HAVE ſeen a large part of the dura mater, and once part of the pia mater oſſified.

CHAPTER. XIV.

Of the cerebrum, cerebellum, medulla oblongata, and medulla ſpinalis.

CEREBRUM is that part of the brain which poſſeſſes all the upper and fore part of the cranium, being ſeparated from the cerebellum by the ſecond proceſs of the dura mater. Its upper ſide is divided into two hemiſpheres, and its lower ſide into four lobes, two anterior and two poſterior, which latter are much the largeſt. At the meeting of the four lobes appears the infundibulum, which ſeems to be a lymphatic, running from the ventricles of the brain into the glandula pituitaria: This gland is ſeated in the ſella turcica. Immediately behind the infundibulum appear two ſmall bodies, named protuberantiæ duæ albæ pone infundibulum. Between the two hemiſpheres of the cerebrum, lower than the circumvolutions, appears a white body, named corpus calloſum. Under the corpus calloſum appear the two lateral or ſuperior ventricles, which are divided into right and left by a very thin membrane, named ſeptum lucidum, which is extended between the corpus calloſum and fornix. The fornix is a medullary body, beginning from the fore part of theſe ventricles, with two ſmall roots which ſoon unite; and running towards the back part, where they divide into parts, called crura fornicis. In the baſis

ſis of theſe two ventricles are four prominences: The two anterior are called (from their inner texture) corpora ſtriata; the other two are named thalami nervorum opticorum. Beyond theſe are two more proceſſes, called nates; and under them, nearer the cerebellum, two called teſtes. Above the nates is ſituated the glandula pinealis, famous for being ſuppoſed, by DES CARTES, the ſeat of the ſoul. And upon the thalami nervorum opticorum are a number of blood-veſſels, glands, and lymphæducts, called plexus choroides. Under the beginning of the fornix is a ſmall hole, called foramen ad radices fornicis, or iter ad infundibulum; and under the middle of the fornix, one called foramen poſterius, which is covered with a valve named membrana, or valvula major; and the ſpace under the two anterior ventricles between the foramina and the cerebellum is the third ventricle.

CEREBELLUM is ſituated under the ſecond proceſs of the dura mater. By dividing this part of the brain length-ways we diſcover more plainly the fourth ventricle, whoſe extremity is called calamus ſcriptorius; here alſo appear two medullary bodies called pedunculi, which are the baſis of the cerebellum. The medullary part in the cerebellum, though it is inmoſt, as in the cerebrum, yet is of a different ſhape, being branched out like a plant.

THE ſubſtance of the brain is diſtinguiſhed into outer and inner: the former is called corticalis, cinerea, or glanduloſa; the latter medullaris, alba, or nervea.

MEDULLA

Medulla oblongata is a medullary continuation of the under part of the cerebrum and cerebellum. It firſt appears in two bodies from the anterior part of the poſterior lobes of the cerebrum, called crura medullæ oblongatæ. The union of theſe crura between the cerebrum and cerebellum is called iſthmus; and immediately beyond this is an eminence named proceſſus annularis.

Medulla spinalis is a production of the medulla oblongata through the great foramen of the ſcull, and through the channel of the ſpine: It enlarges about the laſt vertebræ of the back and firſt of the neck, where the large nerves are given off to the arms: it again enlarges in the loins, where the crural nerves begin; and the lower end of it, with thoſe and other nerves, is called from its reſemblance cauda equina. The coats of this part are the ſame with thoſe of the brain; but the membrane here, which is analogous to the dura mater, is thinner and more connected to the bones, and the tunica arachnoides more conſpicuous.

Wounds in the cerebrum, though very dangerous, are not mortal; but in the cerebellum and medulla oblongata cauſe ſudden death; and in the medulla ſpinalis, loſs of ſenſe in all the parts which receive nerves from below the wound. In perſons that have died lethargic, I have always found the brain full of water; and in children, the brain is always very ſoft and moiſt. In a man, that died of an apoplexy, I found all the veſſels of the brain immo-

immoderately diſtended with blood, and the ventricles and the ſubſtance of the brain full of lymph, the pia mater very much thickened, and adhering ſo very cloſely that the greateſt part of it was ſeparated without breaking.

I HAVE twice ſeen in the cerebrum a ſcirrhous tumor as large as a pullet's egg; and in another body, impoſthumations which poſſeſſed near two thirds of the whole cerebrum. And in a perſon that died with a gutta ſerena, I found all the ventricles of the brain full of lymyh; and the thalami nervorum opticorum and the optic nerves, ere they went out of the ſcull, made flat with the preſſure. And in an old man I found the right optic nerve waſted and black.

CHAPTER XV.

Of the nerves.

" FROM the medullary part of the cere-" brum, cerebellum, and medulla ſpinalis, " a vaſt number of ſmall medullary white fibres " are ſent out, which, at their firſt egreſs, ſeem " eaſily to ſeparate, but as they paſs forward are " ſomewhat more, but ſtill looſely connected, by " the coat which they obtain from the pia mater, " and at laſt piercing the dura mater, are ſtraitly " braced by that membrane which covers them in "their progreſs; whence they become white, firm, "ſtrong cords, and are ſo, well known by the name "of nerves. To theſe coats an infinite number of "veſſels, both arteries and veins, are diſtributed; "ſo that after a nice lucky injection the whole cord "is tinged with the colour of the injected liquor; "but when the fibrils are examined, even with the "beſt microſcope, they appear only like ſo many ſmall "diſtinct threads running parallel, without any ca-"vity obſervable in them, though ſome incautious "obſervers, miſtaking the cut orifices of the arte-"rious and venous veſſels, juſt now mentioned, for "nervous tubes, have affirmed their cavities to be "viſible. The nerves, which if all joined hardly "make a cord of an inch diameter, would ſeem, "from their exerting themſelves every where, to "be diſtributed to each, even the ſmalleſt part of "the body. In their courſe to the places for which "they are deſtined they generally run as ſtrait as the "part over which they are to paſs, and their own "ſafety from external injuries will allow, ſending "off their branches at very acute angles, and con-"ſequently running more parallel than the blood-"veſſels. Their diſtribution is ſeldom different in "the oppoſite ſides of the ſame ſubject, nor in-"deed in any two ſubjects is there conſiderable va-"riety found. Frequently nerves which come out "diſtinct or ſeparate, afterwards conjoin into one "faſciculus, under the ſame common covering; "and though the nervous fibrils probably do not "commu-

" communicate (the reaſon of which opinion ſhall " immediately be given) yet becauſe the coats at " the conjoined part are common, and theſe ſtrong " coats may have great effects on the ſoft pulpy " nerves, it is evident all ſuch will have a conſi- " derable ſympathy with one another, whereof ſe- " veral examples in practice ſhall be inſtanced when " the particular nerves are deſcribed. In ſome parts " where there are ſuch conjunctions, the bulk of " the nerves ſeems much increaſed, and theſe knotty " oval bodies, called by FALLOPIUS corpora oli- " varia, and generally now named ganglions, are " formed. The coats of theſe knots are ſtronger, " thicker, and more muſcular than the whole nerves " which enter into them would ſeem to conſtitute, " while the nervous fibrils paſs through without " any great alteration or change. I do not think " any author has yet made a probable conjecture " of the uſe or deſign of theſe ganglions, whe- " ther they imagine them corcula expellentia, re- " ſervoirs, or elaboratories, neither can I give an " account of their uſe the leaſt ſatisfactory to my- " ſelf.

" FROM undeniable evident experiments, all " anatomiſts are now convinced that to the nerves " we owe all our ſenſation and motion, of which " they are the proper organs; and the ſenſations " in the minuteſt parts being very diſtinct, there- " fore the inſtruments of ſuch ſenſations muſt have " diſtinct origins and courſe to each part. Though "all are agreed as to the effect, yet a hot dispute "has arisen about the manner how it is produced, "viz. whether sensation and motion are occasioned "by a vibration communicated to the nerves, which "these gentlemen suppose entirely solid and tense, "or by a liquid contained and moved in them. "The last of these opinions I rather incline to, for "these reasons, because the nerves proceeding from "the brain bear a great analogy to the excretory "ducts of other glands. Then they are far from "being stretched and tense in order to vibrate. "And what brings the existence of a liquid in their "cavities next to a demonstration, is the experiment "first made by BELLINI, and related by BOHN "and PITCAIRN, which I have often done with "exact good success; it is this: After opening the "thorax of a living dog, catch hold of and compress "the phrenic nerve, immediately the diaphragm "ceases to act; remove the compressing force, that "muscle again contracts; gripe the nerve with one "hand some way above the diaphragm, that sep-"tum is unactive; then with the other hand strip "down the nerve from the first hand to the dia-"phragm, this muscle again contracts; after once "or twice having stripped the nerve thus down "or exhausted the liquid contained in it, the mus-"cle no more acts, squeeze as you will, till the "first hand is taken away or removed higher, and "the nerve stripped, i. e. the liquids in the supe-"rior part of the nerve have free access to the dia-

"phragm,

"phragm, or are forced down to it, when it again "will move. Now if this liquid ſhould be grant- "ed us, I am afraid we ſhall be ſtill as much at "a loſs to account for ſenſation and motion as "ever; and therefore all I ſhall aſſume is what is "founded on experiments, that theſe two actions "do depend on the nerves; that ſenſations are "pleaſant as long as the nerves are only gently af- "fected without any violence offered them; but "as ſoon as any force applied goes beyond this, "and threatens a ſolution of union, it creates that "uneaſy ſenſation, pain: The nerves, their ſource "or their coats being vitiated, either convulſion or "palſy of the muſcles may enſue.

"The nerves are diſtinguiſhed into two claſſes, "of the encephalon and medulla ſpinalis; of the "firſt there are generally ten pair reckoned, of "the laſt thirty. I ſhall deſcribe the nerves in "the ſame order in which they are generally "ranked, though it is not poſſible to proſecute the "diſſection of them after the ſame manner; but "to ſupply this, I ſhall mention alſo the order "wherein they may be all demonſtrated on one "ſubject. When I aſſign the origin of any nerve "from any particular part, I deſire it may be un- "derſtood of that part of the ſurface of the me- "dulla where the nerve firſt appears; for by this "method we ſhall ſhun any diſpute with thoſe au- "thors who trace their riſe too minutely, and per- "haps be leſs liable to miſtake or to deceive our

 "readers.

" readers. Nor ſhall I be over anxious about the " terminations of the minimæ fibrillæ, ſince it is " not poſſible to trace them ad ultimos fines, nor " do I think very neceſſary for explaining any phæ- " nomena, while very often in a multiplicity of " words the whole deſcription comes to be obſcure " or unintelligible.

" Of the ten pair proceeding from the encepha- " lon, the firſt is the olfactory, which in brutes, " juſtly enough, has the name of proceſſus ma- " millares beſtowed on them, being large and hol- " low, and are indeed evidently the two anterior " ventricles of the brain produced; which ſtructure " and the lymph conſtantly found in them, induced " the ancients to believe that they ſerved as emun- " ctories to convey the ſuperabundant mucus from " the cold moiſt brain to the noſe; but in man " they are ſmall, long, and without any cavity, " riſing from that part of the brain where the ca- " rotid arteries are about to enter, and running un- " der the anterior lobes of the brain become a little " larger, till they reach the os cribriforme, into " the foramina of which the ſmall filaments inſi- " nuate themſelves, as upon gently pulling thoſe " nerves, or after having cut them very near the " bone, is evident, and are immediately ſpread on " the membrana narium. Their tender ſtructure " and ſudden expanſion on ſuch a large ſurface, " make it impoſſible to trace them on the mem- " brane of the noſtrils, which has given ſome handle

" to

" to ſeveral authors to deny them the ſtructure or " uſe of nerves.

" THE ſecond are the optic, which ariſe ſingle " from the thalami nervorum opticorum, and then " uniting at the fore part of the cella turcica, they " ſeem to be pretty much blended; afterwards they " divide, and running obliquely forwards, paſs out " at their proper hole of the ſphenoide bone, and " enter the globe of the eye to be expanded into " the membrana retina. From this conjunction of " theſe nerves, authors generally endeavour to ac-" count for our ſeeing objects ſingle, whereas we " have reaſon to believe fiſhes, the chamaleon, &c. " whoſe optic nerves ſimply croſs one another with-" out any ſuch union, do ſee objects alſo ſingle, " ſince they ſo exactly ruſh on their prey; where-" as if thoſe authors aſſertions were true, they " would oftner catch at the ſhadow than the ſub-" ſtance. The blood veſſels running through the " middle of theſe nerves, and the ramifications of " the retina are very obſervable, whence we may " deduce the reaſon of PICARD's experiment of " ſuch objects as fall on the entry of the optic nerve " being loſt to us; and hence alſo an account may " be given of an amauroſis or gutta ſerena.

" THE third pair of nerves firſt appear at the " anterior part of the proceſſus annularis, and go-" ing out at the foramen lacerum are diſtributed to " the globe of the eye; muſculus rectus Fallopii, " attollens, adducens, deprimens, and obliquus mi-

"nor; therefore this pair has juſtly got the name "of motores oculi.

"The fourth pair, which are the ſmalleſt of "any, derive their origins from the anterior lateral "part of the proceſſus annularis, and go out at the "foramina lacera to be intirely ſpent on the muſ-"culi trochleares, or obliqui majores oculorum, to "which muſcles chiefly the rotatory motion of the "eyes in ogling, and the advance of the eyes for-"ward in ſtaring and fury, is owing; for which "reaſon anatomiſts have called theſe nerves pathe-"tici.

"The fifth pair riſe from the ſides of the an-"nular proceſs, and after piercing the dura mater "divide into three branches; the firſt of which is "the ophthalmic, which as it is about to enter the "orbit by the foramen lacerum, ſends off a ſmall "twig that aſſiſts in the formation of the inter-"coſtal, and then the nerve is diſtributed to the "glandula lacrymalis, fat, membranes, and palpe-"bræ of the eye, while it ſends one conſiderable "branch through the orbiter internus anterior hole "to be loſt in the membrana narium, and a ſecond "paſſes the foramen and ſupercilia to ſupply the "muſcles and teguments of the forehead. Hence "we eaſily diſcover what part is affected in that "painful diſeaſe the megrim, when the eye ball "and forehead are racked, and ſuch a heat is felt "within the noſe. Hence alſo we may learn how "the muſcles of reſpiration come to be ſo much "affected

" affected on the application of any acrid irritating " substance to the membrana narium, as to pro- " duce that violent convulsive motion, sneezing. " The second branch of the fifth pair, which may " be called maxillaris superior, passes out through " the foramen rotundum ossis sphenoidis, and im- " mediately gives nerves to the fat under the crota- " phite muscle, and to the palate, sinus sphenoi- " dalis, and nostrils. The remaining trunk insinu- " ating itself into the chanel on the top of the " antrum Highmorianum, to which cavity and to " the teeth of the upper jaw it gives small twigs, " at last comes out at the orbiter externus hole, " and is spent on the musculus orbicularis palpebra- " rum, nose, and upper lip, where some branches " of the seventh pair seem to unite themselves to " the twigs of this. The third branch, or max- " illaris inferior, goes out at the foramen ovale, or " fourth hole of the wedge-like bone, and soon " splitting into a great many branches, is distri- " buted to the musculus crotaphites, masseter, pte- " rygoides, digastricus, buccinator, mylohyoideus, " geniohyoideus, genio-glossus, and basio-glossus, " glandula sublingualis, maxillaris inferior, and " parotis, to the external ear, where it seems to join " the portio dura to the substance of the tongue, " in which it is pretty much confounded with the " ninth pair: from the root of this last branch " the chorda tympani is reflected. The last rami- " fication of this branch which I shall mention, is

" that

" that which enters into the canal of the lower jaw; " furniſhes the teeth there, and comes out at the " chin, on which and the lower lip it is beſtowed; " at this place it is again conjoined to the ſeventh " pair. From this ſhort ſketch of the large fifth " pair of nerves, and by obſerving ſeveral phænomena " which happen to thoſe parts to which they " are diſtributed, we might have a much farther " confirmation of the general doctrine of nerves " delivered, and ſee, at leaſt, the way pathed to a " rational account of theſe phænomena, for reaſoning " on which we ſhould not otherwiſe have the " leaſt ground. We can, for example, from the " chorda tympani and the nerves of the teeth, being " derived from the ſame common trunk, underſtand " how the ſound of any vibrating body " held between our teeth is ſenſible to us, when " another cannot poſſibly hear the leaſt of it. By " the like rule we know why in a violent tooth-ach " the muſcles of the face are ſometimes convulſed; " nor ſhall we be ſurprized to hear one " plagued with the ach in his upper teeth, complain " of a gnawing pain deep ſeated in the bones " of his face, or to ſee his eye-lids much ſwelled, " or the tears trickling down in great abundance; " whereas the lower teeth aching, the ear is pained, " and the ſaliva flows in great quantities. We " may have ſome diſtant views of ſome foundation " in reaſon for the cure of the tooth-ach, by ſtrong " compreſſion of the chin, or by applying bliſters

" behind

" behind the ears, or by burning behind or on the " ear. Among a great many inſtances of the good " effect of the actual cautery in ſuch a caſe, I ſhall " give one which ſeems to me remarkable: I. M. " was ſeized with the tooth-ach, a convulſion of " that whole ſide of his face followed whenever " the pain became acute, or he attempted to ſpeak; " after he had undergone bleeding, purging, ſa- " livation, ſetons, &c. without any benefit, he " was cured by applying a ſmall cauteriſing iron to " the antihelix.

" The ſixth pair of nerves ariſing from the " fore part of the corpora pyramidalia, after piercing " through the dura mater, give off a branch, which " joined with the reflected twig of the ophthalmic " branch of the fifth pair, forms the original of " the intercoſtal, paſſes through the foramen lace- " rum to be ſpent entirely on the muſculus ab- " ductor oculi: Suppoſing this nerve to ſupply ever " ſo little leſs than a due proportion of liquidum " nervoſum, an involuntary ſtrabiſmus will be oc- " caſioned.

" Though the fifth and ſixth pair of nerves " form entirely the beginning of the intercoſtal " before it goes out of the ſcull, yet becauſe ſeve- " ral other nerves contribute towards the forma- " tion of its trunk before it ſends off any branches, " I ſhall superſede the deſcription of it till the ori- " ginal nerves are ſpoke to.

" The

"THE ſeventh pair appears coming out from "the ſide of the root of the annular proceſs, and "entering the meatus auditorius internus, and im-"mediately dividing, one part ſoon loſes its firm "coats, and is expanded on the inmoſt camera of "the ear, while the other paſſing through the aquæ-"ductus Fallopii comes out of the ſcull involved "in all its coats between the ſtyloide and maſtoide "proceſſes; whence we ſee the reaſon of the firſt "being named portio mollis, and the other dura: "This laſt after its exit ſupplies the muſculi obliqui "capitis ſtylohyoidei, ſtylogloſſi, and ſtylopharyn-"gæi, and platyſma myoides, on which, and to "the ſkin of the neck, a great number of its ſmall "filaments run, which are ſometimes cut in open-"ing the jugular vein, whence pain at firſt, and a lit-"tle numbneſs afterwards. The ſuperior branches "of it ſupply the parotid gland, external ear, and "whole ſide of the face as far forwards as the chin. "It is ſaid to communicate thrice with the fifth pair, "and twice with the ſecond vertebra. Whether "may not we hence ſee ſome reaſon why the head "is ſo ſoon moved by the impreſſion of ſound on "our ear?

"THE eighth pair of nerves derive their origin "from the ſide of the baſis of the corpora olivaria, "where their looſe filamentous texture is very con-"ſpicuous; then running to the hole common to "the oſſa temporum and occipitis, they are there "joined by the acceſſorius Williſii, which has its

" beginning from the two or three ſuperior nerves " of the medulla ſpinalis, and mounts upwards " thither, to paſs out with the eighth pair, at that " common foramen juſt now mentioned: Very ſoon " after they, wrapped up in the ſame coat, have " got out of the cranium, the acceſſorius ſeparates " from its companion, and after paſſing through " the middle of the muſculus maſtoideus, is loſt in " the muſculus trapezius and rhomboides ſcapulæ; " while the large trunk, which, from the great " number of branches it ſends off, obtains the name " of vagus, runs ſtrait down the neck, near the " carotid artery, in its courſe giving ſeveral branches " to the larynx: When entered the thorax, it ſplits " into two; the anterior ſerves the pericardium, " ſends branches to join with thoſe of the inter-" coſtal that go to the heart, and then on the right " ſide turns round the ſubclavian, and on the left " round the ductus arterioſus, to mount again up-" wards at the ſide of the œſophagus to be loſt " in the larynx. This recurrent branch it is that " we are earneſtly cautioned to avoid in broncho-" tomy, though by reaſon of its deep ſituation we " are in no hazard of it. If both theſe nerves " were cut, it is probable the voice would not be " entirely loſt as long as the ſuperior branches ſtill " ſupply the larynx. The poſterior branch of the " eighth pair goes along with the œſophagus, and " ſupplies the lungs, the gula, and ſtomach very " plentifully: And as all the nerves beſtowed on " this

"this viſcus enter at the ſuperior orifice of it, the "ſenſation here muſt be very acute; whence HELMONT imagined the mouth of the ſtomach to "be the ſeat of the ſoul. What remains of this "par vagum is adjoined to the intercoſtal immedi- "ately below the diaphragm.

"THE ninth pair appear firſt at the inferior "part of the corpora pyramidalia, and march out "at their proper holes of the occipitis, and after "ſending off ſome nerves to the glandula thyroidea, "and muſculi ſterno-hyoidei, and ſterno-thyroidei, "are loſt in the ſubſtance of the tongue. Authors "have diſputed whether this ninth or the fifth is "the guſtatory nerve; the old opinion in favour of "the ninth is to me moſt probable, becauſe the "fifth is no where elſe employed as an organ of "ſenſation, becauſe the ninth ſeems to penetrate "the ſubſtance of the tongue more, while the "fifth is ſpent on the muſcles.

"THE tenth pair comes out from the beginning "of the medulla ſpinalis, betwixt the os occipitis "and firſt vertebra colli, and is all, except what "goes to the ganglion of the intercoſtal, ſpent on "the muſculi obliqui, and extenſores capitis.

"THE only nerves proceeding from the ence- "phalon not deſcribed, are the reflected branches "of the fifth and ſixth, which indeed are ſo ſmall "and pappy, and hid by the carotid artery as they go "out with it in its crooked canal, as not to be eaſily "traced; but whenever they have eſcaped from the

"os

" os petroſum, they are joined by branches from " the eighth, ninth, tenth, and firſt and ſecond " ſpinal, and the largeſt ganglion of the body is " formed, from which the nerve named now inter- " coſtal, goes out to deſcend down the neck with " the carotid, ſupplying in its courſe the muſculi " flexores of the head and neck, and communicating " with the cervical nerves. As the intercoſtal is a- " bout to enter the thorax, it again forms a ganglion, " from which the nerves to the trachea arteria and " the heart are ſupplied, which join with the " branches of the eighth, and paſs between the " two large arteries and auricles to the ſubſtance of " that muſcle. Now let any one conſider the " egreſs of the intercoſtal, and cloſe courſe of it " and the eighth with the carotid artery, and this " manner of entry of the cardiac nerves, ſurely the " alternate conſtriction and relaxation of the heart " will appear neceſſarily depending on the diſpoſi- " tion of theſe organs of motion, the nerves. The " intercoſtal after this runs down on the ſide of the " vertebræ thoracis, having additional nerves con- " ſtantly ſent to it from between theſe vertebræ, " till it paſs through its own proper hole of the " diaphragm; whence it again forms another gan- " glion cloſe by the glandulæ renales, into which " the eighth pair enter. From ſuch a knot on each " ſide, the nerves of the guts, liver, ſpleen, pan- " creas, and kidneys are derived; nay the extremi- " ty of this nerve is ſent down to the pelvis to ſup-

" ply

" ply the parts there. Hence the great ſympathy " of theſe parts may be eaſily deduced, and a rea- " ſon may be given of the violent vomiting that " commonly attends a nephritis, and of the belch- " ing, cholic, and ſtomach-achs, which often enſue " on the obſtructions of the menſtrua.

" Before I proceed to the ſpinal nerves, I " ſhall ſet down the order in which theſe nerves " already deſcribed, are to be diſſected, in order to " demonſtrate them all in one ſubject, but to them " muſt aſſume the three firſt cervical nerves, the " reaſon of which will be evident afterwards.

" Portio dura septimi, frontalis quinti, " facialis quinti, mentalis quinti, ſpinalis ſecundus, " ſpinalis primus, olfactorius, ophthalmicus quinti, " motorius oculi, patheticus ſextus, opticus, max- " illaris inferior quinti, maxillaris ſuperior quinti, " acceſſorius Williſii, nonus, decimus, octavus in- " tercoſtalis, portio mollis ſeptimi.

" The thirty pair of nerves proceeding from the " medulla ſpinalis are generally divided into four " ſpecies; of the neck ſeven, of the back twelve, " of the loins five, and of the os ſacrum ſix. Now " as the medulla ſpinalis has none of theſe inequa- " lities ſo obſervable on the medulla oblongata " encephali, the riſe of the nerves is not ſo accu- " rately deſcribed, being only determined by the " bones through which they paſs.

" The firſt cervical goes out between the firſt " and ſecond vertebra, and, after ſending off branches " that

"that communicate with the tenth and fecond "vertebrale, is fpent on the mufculus flexus colli, "fplenius, complexus, and teguments of the occi-"pitis.

"The fecond cervical communicates with the "ninth, and with the firft and third of the neck, "and then is diftributed to the teguments of the "neck and fide of the head, and to the glandula "parotis and external ear, where it joins with the "portio dura.

"The third of the neck paffes out between the "third and fourth vertebra, foon communicating "with the fecond, and fending down a large branch, "which being joined by another from the fourth, "forms the phrenic nerve that runs along the pe-"ricardium to be loft in the diaphragm. In this "courfe the right phrenic is obliged to make a fmall "turn round that part of the pericardium which "covers the apex of the heart. Hence it is that "fuch as have ftrong palpitations of the heart, feel "a pungent acute pain immediately above the right "orifice of the ftomach. The other branches of "this third cervical are diftributed to the mufculus "trapezius and deltoides, and to the teguments on "the top of the fhoulder; which, with the de-"fcription of the eighth pair, leads us evidently to "the reafons of the divine Hippocrates's ob-"fervation, that an inflammation of the liver is "generally attended with a hiccough, and a fuppu-"ration of that vifcus, with a violent pain on the "top of the ſhoulder. However, we are not hence "to conclude ſo generally, as I have obſerved phy-"ſicians frequently do, that if the hypochondria are "affected, and this pain of the ſhoulder is felt, "therefore the liver is ſuppurated; for any other "cauſe ſtimulating or ſtretching the nerves, ſuch as "inflammation, wounds, ſcirrhous or ſteatomatous "tumors, &c. may produce the ſame effect.

"THE fourth cervical, after ſending off that "branch which joins with the third to form the "phrenic, runs ſtrait to the axilla, where it meets "with the fifth, ſixth, and ſeventh cervicals, and "firſt dorſal that eſcape in the interſtices of the "muſculi ſcaleni; and all of them are ſo often "conjoined and blended, after they have given off "nerves to the muſcles of the neck, ſcapula, arm, "and thorax, and to the teguments, that when the "ſeveral ramifications go off in the axilla to the "different parts of the ſuperior extremity, it is im-"poſſible to determine which of them the branches "belong to. The conſiderable branches into which "they are divided, are ſix; theſe I ſhall preſume "to give proper diſtinguiſhing names to, by which "the deſcription will be leſs confuſed, and the "young anatomiſt's memory better aſſiſted to retain "what is ſo difficult to repreſent in words.

"1. CUTANEUS runs down the fore-part of "the arm, and ſerves the teguments, as far as "the palm of the hand and fingers.

"2. MUSCULO-

"2. MUSCULO-CUTANEUS, or PERFORANS "CASSERII, passes through the musculus coraco-"brachialis, and after supplying the biceps and "brachiæus internus, is spent on the teguments of "the back of the cubitus and hand.

"3. MUSCULARIS, that runs down the fore-"part of the arm to be lost in the musculi flexores, "carpi, digitorum, &c.

"4. ULNARIS, which supplies the extensores "cubiti, and teguments of the elbow, and then "passing through the sinuosity at the back of the "external condyle of the humerus, runs along the "ulna, where it gives twigs to the teguments and "neighbouring muscles; at length is lost in the "back of the hand, musculi interossei, and lumbri-"cales in the little finger, and side of the ring "finger next to this. The course of this nerve is "sufficiently felt when we lean on our elbow, by "the insensibility and prickling pain in the parts "to which it is distributed.

"5. RADIALIS goes down the fore-part of the "arm, near the radius, bestowing branches in its "progress on the circumjacent muscles, and at the "ligamentum annulare carpi splitting, is sent to the "thumb, fore finger, middle finger, and half of "the ring finger, and to the back of the hand.

"6. ARTICULARIS runs almost round the top "of the os humeri, and serves the musculi exten-"sores cubiti, retractores, and elevatores humeri.

"By a ſtrong and continued preſſure on theſe
" nerves, by crutches or any ſuch hard ſubſtance,
" a palſy and atrophy of the arm may be occa-
" ſioned.

"The twelve dorſal nerves all communicate
" with one another; as ſoon as they make their
" way out betwixt the vertebræ, each of them
" gives a poſterior branch to the muſculi erectores
" trunci corporis; the firſt, after having ſent off
" the brachial nerve, already deſcribed, is, after the
" ſame manner with the ſucceeding eight, be-
" ſtowed on the pleura and intercoſtal muſcles;
" the tenth and eleventh are moſt of them ſent to
" the abdominal muſcles; the twelfth communi-
" cates with the firſt lumbar, and is beſtowed on the
" muſculus quadratus lumbalis and iliacus internus.

"The fifth lumbar alſo communicates and gives
" poſterior branches; the firſt ſends ſeveral branches
" to the abdominal muſcles, and pſoas and iliacus,
" while others go from it to the teguments and
" muſcles on the ſuperior and anterior part of the
" thigh, and the main trunk of it is loſt in the
" crural. The ſecond paſſes through the pſoas
" muſcle, and is diſtributed much as the former.
" The third is loſt in the muſculus pectineus.
" Branches proceeding from the firſt, ſecond, and
" third, make up one trunk, which runs along the
" anterior part of the pelvis, and ſlipping through a
" ſmall ſinuoſity in the anterior part of the foramen
" magnum oſſis iſchii, is ſpent in the muſculus

"triceps. This nerve is commonly known by "the name of obturator, or posterior crural nerve. "By the union of branches from the first, second, "third, and fourth lumbar nerves, the anterior "crural nerve is formed, which running along the "musculus psoas, escapes with the large blood-"vessels out of the abdomen below the tendinous "arcade of its muscles, and is distributed to the "muscles and teguments on the fore-part of the "thigh: One branch of this crural nerve accom-"panies the vena saphena as far as the ancle. Now "let us imagine the situation of the kidney upon, "and the course of the ureter over these nerves, "and we shall not be surprized, that in a nephri-"tis the trunk of the body cannot be raised erect "without great pain; that the thigh loses of its "sensibility, and that it is drawn forwards. The "remainder of the fourth and the fifth lumbar "nerves join with the first, second, and third that "proceed from the os sacrum: These five, when "united, constitute the largest nerve of the body, "so well known by the name of the sciatic, or "ischiatic nerve, which seems to be bigger, in pro-"portion to the part for the use of which it is, "than the nerves of any other part are; the de-"sign of which may be to afford sufficient strength "to the muscles of the lower extremity, for ex-"erting a force superior to what is required in any "other part of the body. When this nerve is any "way obstructed, we see how unable we are to

" support ourselves, or to walk. The sciatic nerve " then goes out at the large hollow, behind the " great tubercle of the os ischium, and passing " over the quadrigemini muscles, runs down the " posterior part of the thigh, giving off, every " where as it goes, nerves to the teguments and " muscles of the thigh and leg. At the ham it " splits into two; the smaller mounts over the fi- " bula, and serving the musculi peronei, flexores " pedis, and extensores digitorum, is continued to " the toes along the broad of the foot, while the " larger trunk sinks under the musculi gemelli, and " then divides; one is spent on the muscles at the " back of the leg and teguments, while the other " is continued by the inner ancle to the foot, and " then subdivides; one branch is distributed after " the same manner as the ulnaris, and the other as " the radialis in the hand.

" THE other nerves that come out of the os " sacrum, are sent to the organs of generation, " musculi levatores ani, and obturatores.

" THESE nerves of the medulla spinalis may all " be dissected and demonstrated in the same order " in which they are described." For this accurate description of the nerves I am obliged to Mr. MONRO.

THE nerves seem, when examined with a microscope, to be bundles of strait fibres not communicating with one another: And I am inclined to think, that every the minutest nerve, terminating in any part, is a diſtinct cord from its origin in the brain or ſpinal marrow; or elſe I do not ſee how they could produce diſtinct ſenſations in every part; and the diſtinct points of ſenſation throughout the body are ſo numerous, that the whole body of nerves (which taken together would not make a cord of an inch diameter) muſt be divided into ſuch a number, to afford one for every part that has a diſtinct ſenſation, that ſurely ſuch a nerve would be too ſmall to be ſeen by the beſt microſcope. They all paſs in as direct courſes to the places they ſerve, as is poſſible, never ſeparating nor joining with one another but at very acute angles; unleſs where they unite in thoſe knots which are called ganglions, the uſe of which I do not pretend to know; they make what appears to be a communication of moſt of the nerves on the ſame ſide, but never join nerves on oppoſite ſides.

That the nerves are inſtruments of ſenſation, is clearly proved from experiments, but how they convey thoſe ſenſations to the brain, is matter of diſpute. The moſt general opinion is, that they are tubes to contain animal ſpirits, by whoſe motions theſe ſenſations are conveyed: And diligent enquiry has been made to diſcover their cavities, but hitherto in vain; and if each nerve is diſtinct from its origin, as I have endeavoured to ſhew, and too ſmall to be the object of the beſt microſcope, I do not ſee how ſuch cavities are like to be diſco-

 vered.

vered. Neverthelefs nerves may be tubes, and poffibly a fluid, whofe cohefion is very little, and whofe parts, no finer than light, may move freely in them. Thofe who deny animal fpirits in the nerves, fuppofe that the fenfation is conveyed by a vibration. To which it is objected, that they are flack, moift, and furrounded with foft parts, and are therefore unfit for vibrations, as indeed they are for fuch as are made on the ftrings of a mufical inftrument; but the minuteft vibrations, fuch as they cannot be without, may, for aught we know, be as fufficient for this end, as the impulfe of light upon the retina is for the fenfe of feeing. So that perhaps fenfations may be conveyed either, or both ways. However, it being ufually taken for granted, that it muft be one of thefe ways at leaft, the advocates for each have rather endeavoured to fupport their opinions by arguments againft the probability of the other, than by reafons offered for their own.

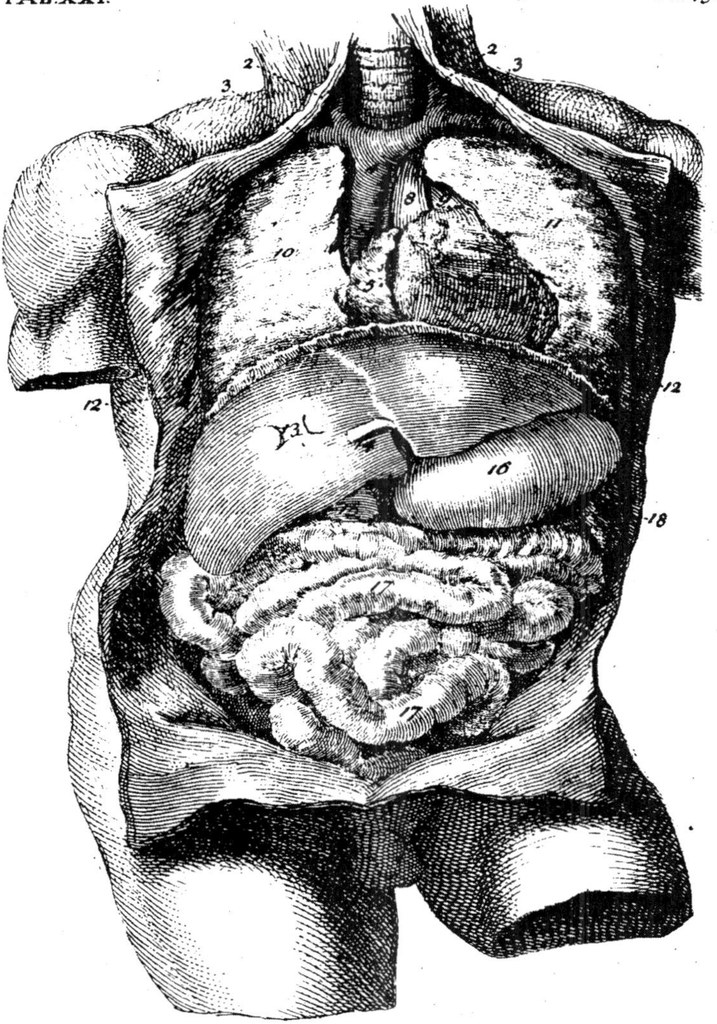
2
3
2
3
8
9
10
11
12
12
16
18
17
17

TAB. XXI.

1 Larynx.
2 The internal jugular vein.
3 The ſubclavian vein.
4 Cava deſcendens.
5 The right auricle of the heart.
6 The right ventricle.
7 Part of the left ventricle.
8 Aorta aſcendens.
9 Arteria pulmonalis.
10 The right lobe of the lungs, part of which is cut off to ſhew the great blood-veſſels.
11 The left lobe of the lungs.
12 The diaphragm.
13 The liver.
14 The ligamentum rotundum.
15 The gall bladder.
16 The ſtomach, preſſed by the liver toward the left-ſide.
17 The ſmall guts.
18 The ſpleen.

TAB. XXII.

1 The under ſide of the liver.
2 Ligamentum rotundum.
3 The gall-bladder.
4 The pancreas.
5 The ſpleen.
6 The kidney.
7 Aorta deſcendens.
8 Vena cava aſcendens.
9 The emulgent vein.
10 A probe under the ſpermatic veſſels and the arteria meſenterica inferior, and over the ureters.
11 The ureter.
12 The iliac veſſels.
13 The rectum inteſtinum.
14 The bladder of urine.

TAB. XXIII.

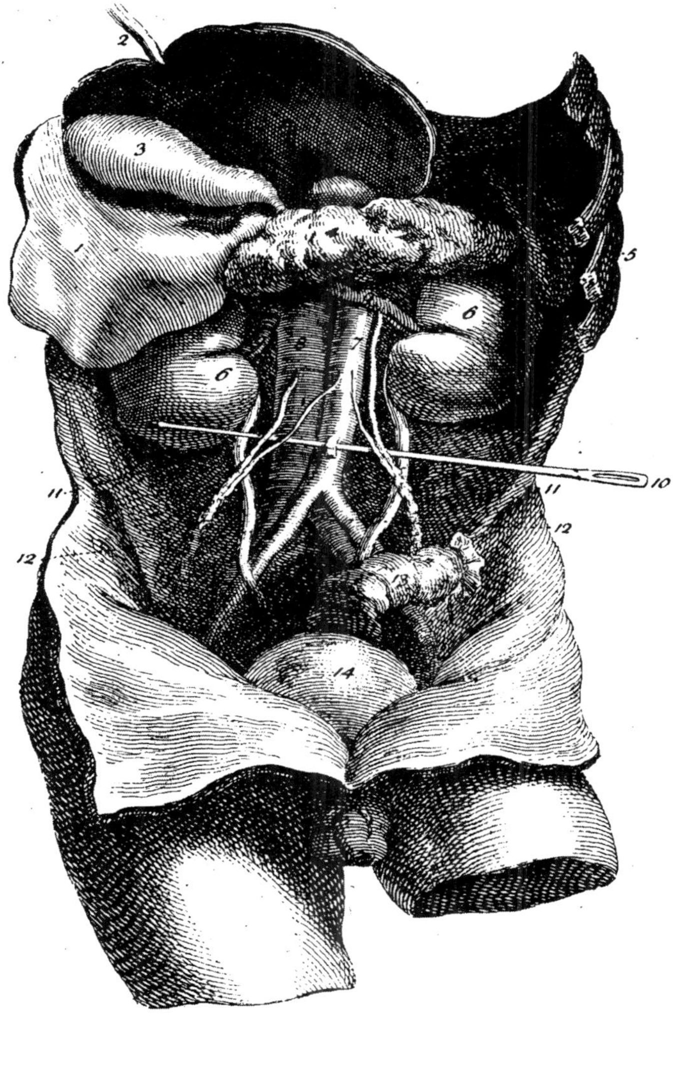

2
3
1
4
5
6
6
8
7
10
11
11
12
12
13
14

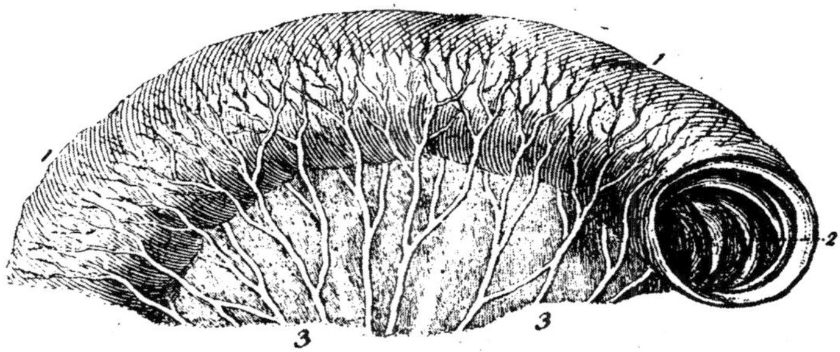
1
1
2
3
3

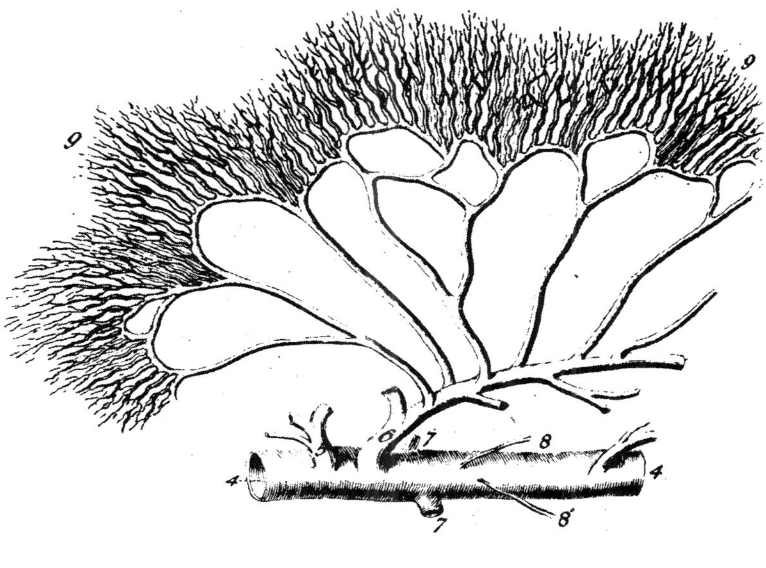
9
9
6
7
8
4
4
7
8

TAB. XXIII.

1 Part of the inteſtinum jejunum.
2 The valvulæ conniventes, as they appear in a dried preparation.
3 The venæ lacteæ ariſing from the gut, and paſſing through part of the meſentery.
4 Part of the deſcending aorta.
5 Arteria cœliaca.
6 Meſenterica ſuperior.
7 Emulgentes.
8 Spermaticæ.
9 Some of the branches of the meſenterica inferior that are beſtowed upon the guts.

TAB. XXIV.

TAB. XXIV.

1 Extreme branches of the vena porta, as they arise from the guts.

2 All the branches of the vena porta, united before it enters the liver.

3 The branches of the vena porta, as they are distributed in the liver.

TAB. XXV.

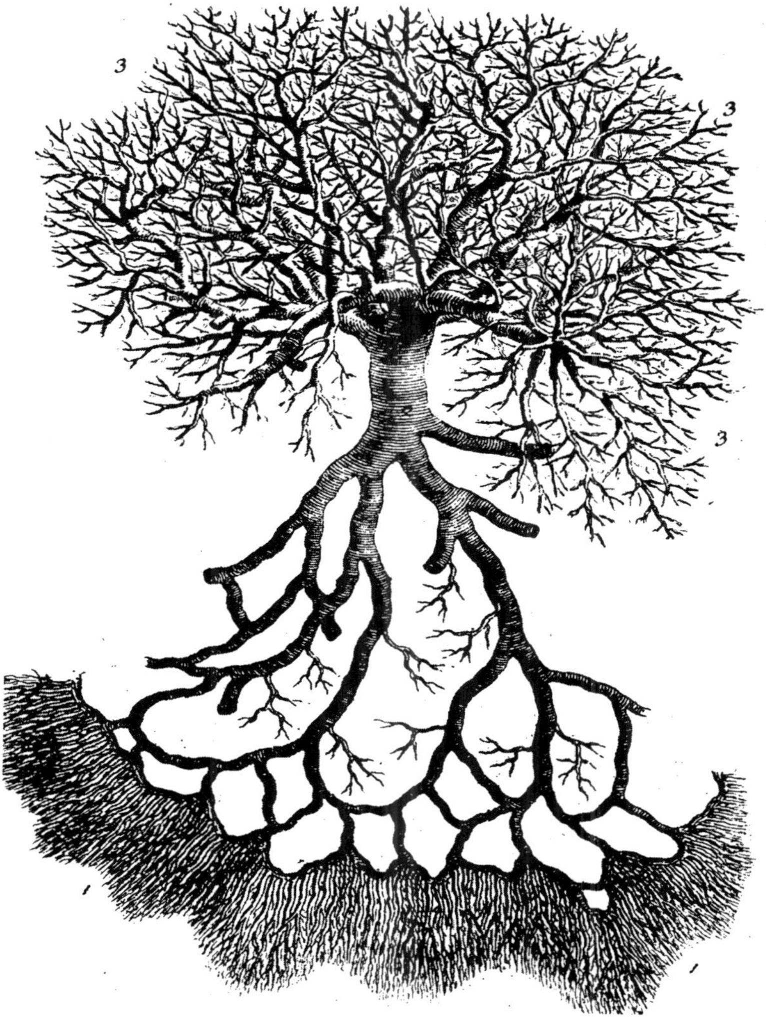
3
3
3
1
1

TAB. XXV.

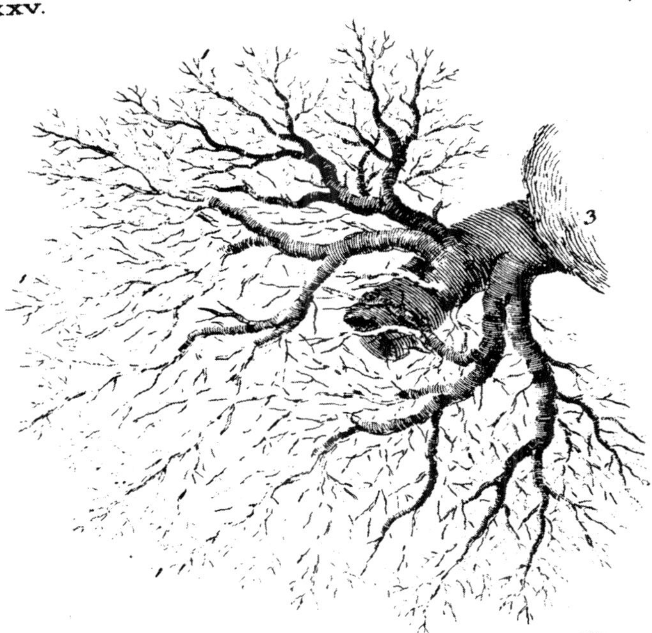

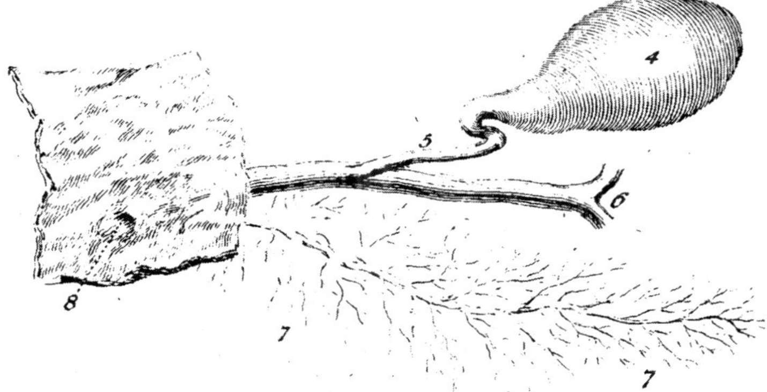

TAB. XXV.

1 Branches of the vena cava in the liver.
2 Part of the vena cava aſcendens.
3 Part of the right auricle.
4 Cyſtis hepaticus.
5 Ductus cyſticus.
6 Ductus hepaticus.
7 Ductus pancreaticus.
8 The entrance of the ductus communis into the duodenum.

TAB. XXVI.

TAB. XXVI.

1 The left ſubclavian vein.
2 The internal jugular.
3 Part of the vena azygos.
4 Part of the deſcending aorta.
5 The ſubclavian artery.
6 Some of the lacteals entering the receptaculum chyli.
7 Some lymphatics entering the receptaculum chyli.
8,9 Ductus thoracicus.
10 The entrance of the thoracic duct into the ſubclavian vein.

TAB. XXVII.

TAB. XXVI.

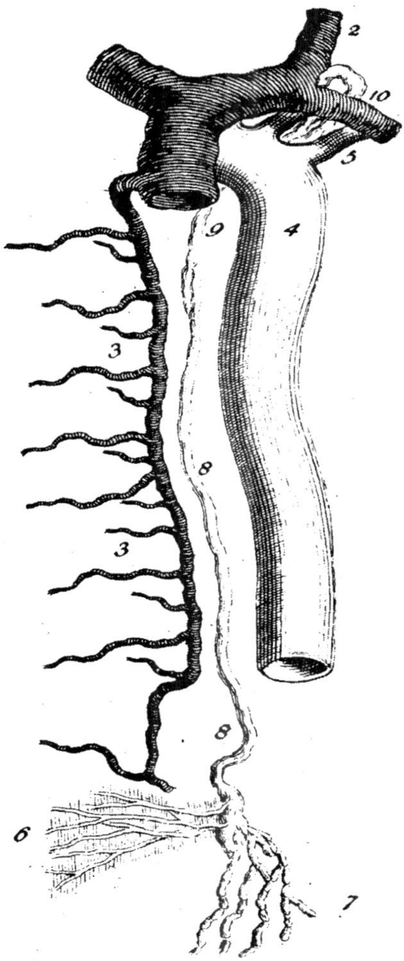

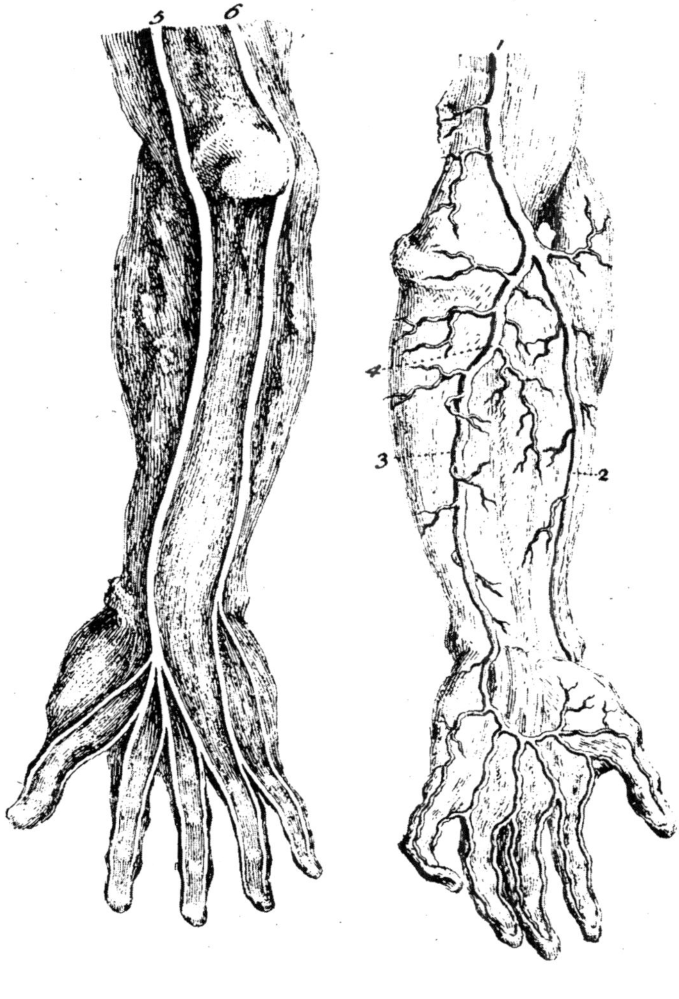
5
6
1
4
3
2

TAB. XXVII.

1 The humeral artery.
2 Cubitalis ſuperior.
3 Cubitalis inferior, which ends in the hand and the fingers, and communicates with the cubitalis ſuperior, under the muſcles of the thumb.
4 The place where the cubitalis media is given off.
5 The ſuperior cubital nerve.
6 The inferior cubital nerve, which paſſes under the inner extuberance of the os humeri; both theſe nerves give off branches as they paſs, and end in the thumb and fingers.

TAB. XXVIII.

T A B. XXVIII.

1 Part of the biceps flexor cubiti.

2 The faſcia tendinoſa from that muſcle, which is liable to be pricked in bleeding in the baſilic vein.

3 The humeral artery, on each ſide of which is a large vein.

4 Vena cephalica.

5 Mediana.

6 Baſilica.

7 A tumor formed in the centre of the cubital nerve, a little above the bend of the arm; it was of the cyſtic kind, but contained a tranſparent jelly; the filaments of the nerve were divided and ran over its ſurface. This tumor occaſioned a great numbneſs in all the parts that nerve leads to, and exceſſive pain upon the leaſt touch or motion. This operation was done but a few weeks ſince, the pain is entirely ceaſed, the numbneſs a little increaſed, and the limb, as yet, not waſted.

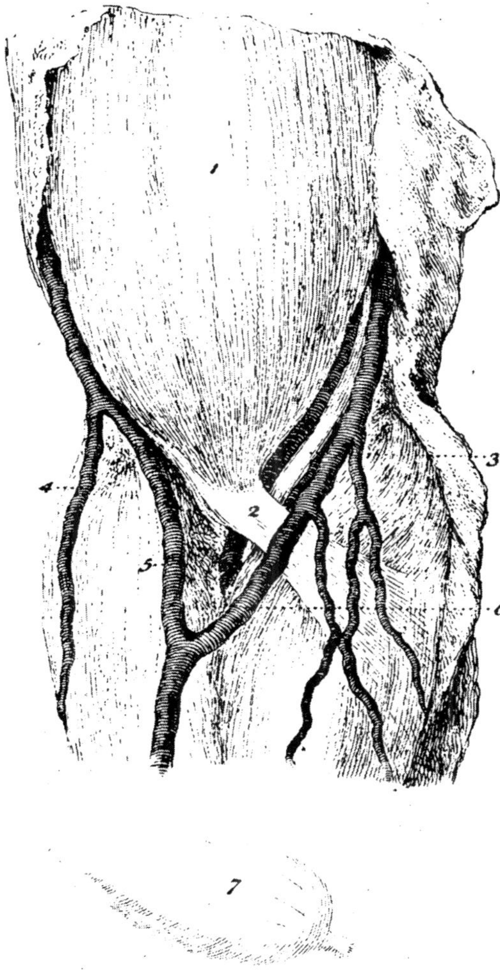
1
2
3
4
5
6
7

TAB. XXIX.

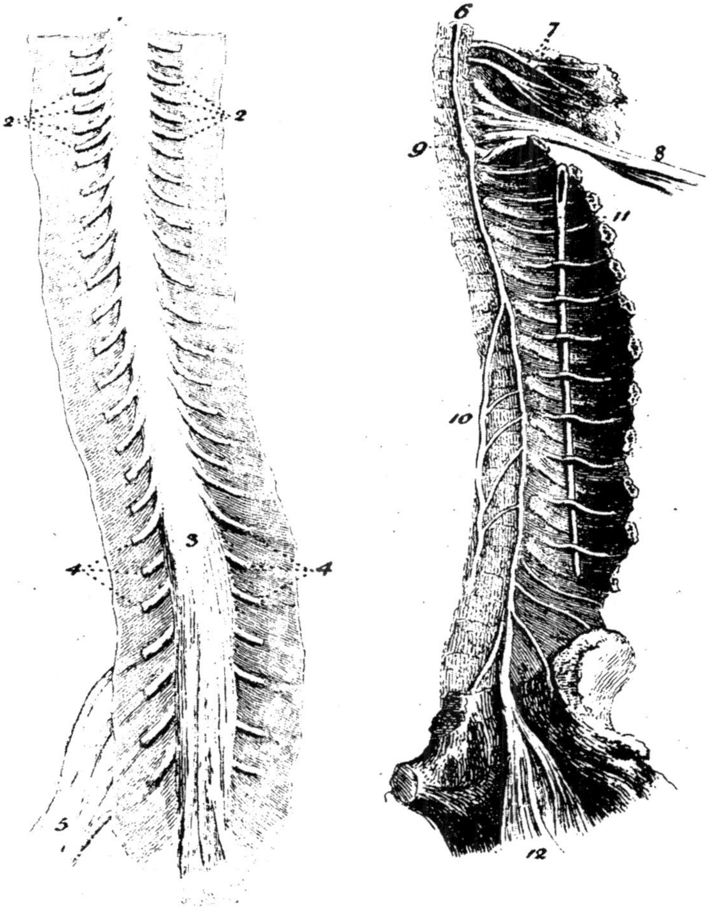

TAB. XXIX.

1 The medulla ſpinalis, from whence ariſe the nerves that paſs out between the vertebræ.
2 The brachial nerves.
3 The beginning of the cauda equina.
4 The anterior crural nerves.
5 The poſterior crural nerves.
6 The deſcending intercoſtal.
7 Nerves of the neck.
8 The brachial nerves.
9 A ganglion in the deſcending intercoſtal nerve.
10 Branches from the intercoſtal nerve to the viſcera.
11 A probe paſſed under ſome of the intercoſtal nerves that paſs out between the ribs.
12 The anterior crural nerves.

TAB. XXX.

1 The animalculæ in ſemine maſculino, as they appeared in a microſcope, in a ſpace as ſmall as a pin's head.

2 The circulation of the blood in a fiſh's tail, as it appeared in a microſcope.

3 An artery, as it is ſpread in a membrane.

4 A vein, as it is ſpread in a membrane.

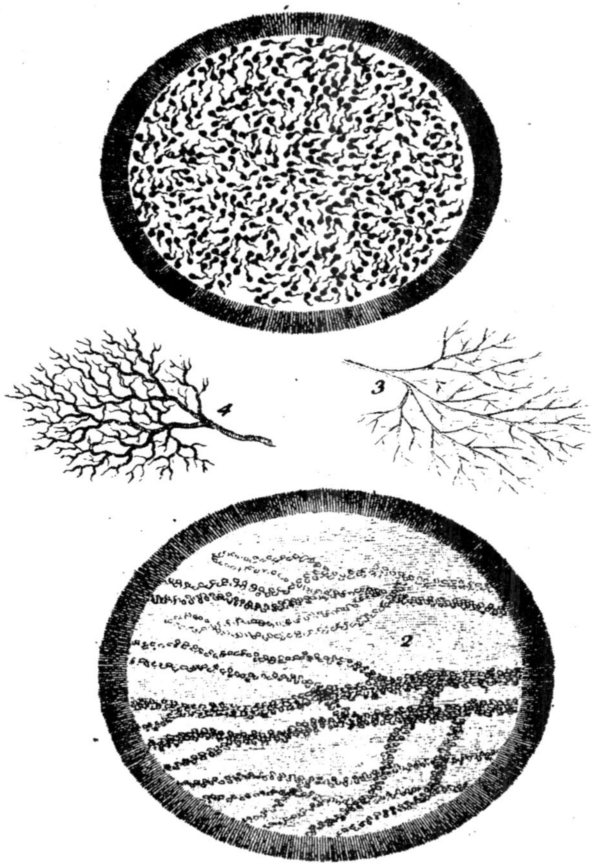
4
3
2

THE ANATOMY OF THE Human Body.

BOOK IV.

CHAPTER I.

Of the urinary and genital parts of men, together with the glandulæ renales.

THE urinary parts are the kidneys with their veſſels and bladder of urine.

THE kidneys of men are like thoſe of hogs; the two weigh about twelve ounces; they are ſeated towards the upper part of the loins upon the two laſt ribs; the right under the liver, and a little lower than the other, and the left under the ſpleen. Their uſe is to ſeparate the urine from the blood, which is brought thither for that purpoſe by by the emulgent arteries; and what remains from the ſecretion, is returned by the emulgent veins, while the urine ſecreted is carried off through the ureters to the bladder. I have, in three different ſubjects, taken ſtones out of the loins, which had made their way from the kidneys through the muſcles to the common integuments, where, upon opening the ſkin only, the ſtones appeared with a quantity of matter and urine. We have heard of operators who have cut for the ſtone in the kidneys; but I will venture to affirm, that thoſe caſes were no other than theſe, tho' unfairly related.

THE ureters are tubes about the bigneſs of gooſe-quills, and about a foot long; they ariſe from the hollow ſide of the kidneys, and end in the bladder near its neck, running obliquely for the ſpace of an inch between its coats; which manner of entering is to them as valves. The beginning of the ureters in the kidneys are the tubuli urinarii, which joining, form the pelvis in each kidney. Between the tubuli urinarii, authors have remarked ſmall papillæ; and the parts which are diſtinguiſhed by a clearer colour, they call glandulæ.

THE bladder of urine is ſeated in a duplicature of the peritonæum in the lower part of the pelvis of the abdomen; its ſhape is orbicular, and its coats are the ſame with thoſe of the guts and other hollow muſcles already deſcribed; viz. an external membranous, a middle muſcular, which is the muſculus detruſor urinæ, and an inner membranous

coat,

coat, exceeding ſenſible, as is fully ſhewn in the caſes of the ſtone and gravel. The uſe of this nice ſenſe is to make it capable of that uneaſineſs which excites animals to exclude their water, when the bladder is extended. This ſenſe is ſo delicate, that no fluid but natural urine can be long endured, even pale urine, or urine with matter in it, in a degree excite the ſymptoms of the ſtone, and force the perſon to void the urine. Sometimes much matter from the kidneys will excite vehement ſymptoms; and this being found in the urine, and the pain being obſerved in the bladder only, the kidneys having little ſenſe of pain, it is uſually accounted for from ulcers in the bladder, which I have never found one inſtance of in all the numbers that I have opened in this caſe. Indeed the bladder is ſometimes ulcerated, but that deſtroying part of the inner coat, the others ſtretch and ulcerate till the urine burſts through into the cellular membrane of the peritonæum, and cauſe a moſt miſerable death. This caſe is very rare in men, and much more ſo in women. I have ſeen cancerous ulcers open the bladder into the uterus, but theſe, I think, have begun in the uterus. All theſe caſes have ſymptoms like the ſtone; and not theſe only, but all diſeaſes of the uterus which diſturb the bladder, and even impoſtumations or tumors that preſs upon the bladder, all give the ſame ſymptoms with the ſtone; except that of a needleſs diſpoſition to ſtool at the time of making water. Some anatomiſts, not thinking how ſoon fluids taken into the ſtomach, and not retained there by being mixed with ſolids, may paſs into the blood, as the effects from drinking ſtrong liquors or laudanum, or drinking without eating when we are hot, ſufficiently ſhew; and alſo not conſidering the ſhortneſs of the courſe from the ſtomach to the kidneys this way, together with the ſize of the emulgent arteries, and the velocity of the blood in them, have imagined and affirmed, that there muſt be ſome more immediate courſe from the ſtomach or guts to the bladder; and not conſidering either how ſuch a courſe would have interrupted one great end in the animal œconomy, or that veſſels fit to fill the bladder faſter than the ureters, muſt have been too large to be concealed; nor, which proves it beyond contradiction, that the bladder is empty when the kidneys ceaſe to do their office; which is frequently taken for a ſuppreſſion of urine in the bladder. If in this laſt caſe, upon making a preſſure on the region of the bladder, the patient does not feel great pain, it is ſcarce worth while to paſs a catheter to ſearch for urine. In ſuppreſſions of urine, whether merely inflammatory, or from the gout, or from an inflamed ſtricture in the urethra, I have found nothing ſo effectual as bleeding, and purging. In a ſanguine large man, where the penis was too much inflamed to ſuffer the catheter to paſs, I took away three times twenty four ounces of blood, and gave a purging clyſter, and two ſtrong purges, all within the ſpace of twenty hours, which ſaved

the

the patient, and delivered him from exceſſive torment. Such practice may ſeem very ſevere, but in this caſe no time is to be loſt; if the urine can be drawn off, this method of cure is ſtill the ſame, but to be practiſed in a gentler manner.

GLANDULÆ RENALES are two glands ſeated immediately above the kidneys, of no certain figure, nor do we know their uſe; but always paint and deſcribe them with the urinary parts, becauſe of their ſituation: In a very young fœtus they are larger than the kidneys, and in an adult but a little larger than in a fœtus. They receive a great many ſmall arteries, and return each of them one or two veins. In their inſide is a ſmall ſinus, tinctured with a ſooty-coloured liquor.

THE teſtes are ſeated in the ſcrotum; their office is to ſeparate the ſeed from the blood; they are ſaid to have four coats, two common, and two proper. The common are the outer ſkin and a looſe membrane immediately underneath, called dartos. The firſt of the proper is the proceſſus vaginalis; it is continued from the peritonæum to the teſticle, which it encloſes with all its veſſels, but is divided by a ſeptum, or an adheſion immediately above the teſticle, ſo that no liquor can paſs out of that part of this membrane, which encloſes the ſpermatic veſſels, into that which encloſes the teſticle. Large quantities of water are ſometimes found in either or both of theſe cavities, which diſeaſe is eaſily remedied by a puncture with a lancet; but rarely cured without opening the cavity where the water is contained, as in ſinuous ulcers. This I have done, and ſeen done ſeveral times, but never thought the cure worth the trouble and pain the patient underwent. The true hernia aquoſa is from the abdomen, which either extends the peritonæum into the ſcrotum, or breaks it, and then forms a new membrane which thickens as it extends, as in aneuriſms and atheromatous tumors. This may be decided by an injection, which will ſhew by the arteries that nouriſh it, whether it is a production from the peritonæum, or a new membranous bag formed in the ſcrotum: However, the dropſy in this ciſt, for ſuch it properly is, rarely admits of more than a palliative cure by puncture or tapping, like the dropſy of the abdomen, and this with ſome difficulty, becauſe the omentum uſually, and ſometimes the gut, deſcends with it. The other proper coat is the albuginea, which is very ſtrong, immediately incloſing the teſticles. The teſticles of a rat may be unravelled into diſtinct veſſels; and the texture of the teſticles of other animals appear to be the ſame, but their veſſels are too tender, or cohere too much to be ſo ſeparated. The teſticles receive each one artery from the aorta, a little below the emulgents, which, unlike all other arteries, ariſe ſmall, and dilate in their progreſs, that the velocity of the blood may be ſufficiently abated for the ſecretion of ſo viſcid a fluid as the ſeed. The right teſticle returns its vein into the cava, and the left

left into the emulgent vein on the ſame ſide, both becauſe it is the readieſt courſe, and becauſe, as authors ſay, this ſpermatic vein would have been obſtructed by the pulſe of the aorta, if it had croſſed that veſſel to go to the cava.

A GENTLEMAN, whom I caſtrated many years ſince, who truſted too much to his own reſolution, and refuſing to have any one preſent to hold him, except my aſſiſtant, during the operation, moved ſo much, that the ligature which tied all the veſſels with the proceſs together, ſlipt, and only tied the proceſs over the ends of the veſſels: Which being perceived ſoon after the operation, I cut the ligature, and took out the extravaſated blood, and tied the artery alone, which gave but little pain, and it digeſted off in a week's time, and the wound being afterwards ſtiched, though the teſticle weighed a pound, it was perfectly well in five weeks; which is in leſs time than the ligature ſometimes requires to be digeſted off, when the proceſs and all the veſſels are tied together. However, if this caſe is not ſufficient to recommend doing this operation by tying the artery only, it may be ſufficient to recommend extraordinary care in doing of it the uſual way; for if the blood had found an eaſy paſſage into the abdomen, the patient might have bled to death.

ON the upper part of the teſticles, are hard bodies called epididymi; which are evidently the beginning of the vaſa deferentia. I have unravelled them

them backward, in single vessels, and then into more and smaller, like the excretory vessels of other glands.

Vasa deferentia are excretory ducts to carry the elaborated seed into the vesiculæ seminales. They pass from the epididymi of the testicles, together with the blood-vessels, till they have entered the muscles of the abdomen, and then they pass under the peritonæum, directly through the pelvis, to the vesiculæ seminales.

Vesiculæ seminales are two bodies that appear like vesicles; they are seated under the bladder of urine, near its neck; they may be each of them unfolded into one single duct, which discharges into the urethra, by the sides of the rostrum gallinaginis, which is an eminence in the underside of the urethra near the neck of the bladder. In these vesicles, or ducts, the seed is reposited against the time of coition; but in dogs there are no such vesicles, therefore nature has contrived a large bulb in their penis, which keeps them coupled, seemingly against their inclinations, till the seed can arrive from the testicles. The seed passes from these vesicles in men, and even from the vasa deferentia, in time of coition, through the prostate glands into the urethra, as in those animals that have no vesiculæ seminales, for when the ducts into the urethra are distended, that is the direct course from the vasa deferentia, as well as from the vesiculæ seminales.

Prostatæ

Prostatæ are two glands, or rather one, about the ſize of a nutmeg: They lie between the veſiculæ ſeminales and penis, under the oſſa pubis almoſt within the pelvis of the abdomen. They ſeparate a limpid glutinous humour which is carried into the urethra by ſeveral ducts, which enter near thoſe of the proſtatæ. This liquor ſeems to be deſigned to be mixed with the ſeed in the urethra, in the time of coition, to make it flow more eaſily. If the venereal infection reaches the proſtate glands, it will ſometimes make large abſceſſes, which are apt to form ſinuſes, and even make a paſſage into the bladder. Upon the firſt attack of this diſeaſe, I have prevented all this miſchief, by taking off the external ſkin by inciſion, as far as the hardneſs of the tumour extended, which draining very plentifully, the tumour has ſubſided, and the patient been eaſily cured; but this caſe once becoming fiſtulous, is very difficult indeed. It often is cured by opening the ſinuſes and conſuming the diſeaſed parts by eſcarotics; but a much better and eaſier way, which I have often done, is to cut out all the fiſtulous and diſeaſed parts at once.

Penis; its ſhape, ſituation, and uſe, need no deſcription. It begins with two bodies named crura, from the oſſa iſchia, which unite under the oſſa pubis, and are there ſtrongly connected by a ligament. In its under part is the urethra, through which both the urine and ſeed paſs; its fore-

fore-part is called glans, the loose skin which covers it, præputium, and the strait part of that skin on the under side, frænum. The urethra is lined with a membrane filled with small glands that separate a mucus, that defends it from the acrimony of the urine. These glands are largest nearest the bladder. Mr. COWPER describes three large glands of the urethra, which he discovered; two of which are seated on the sides of the urethra, near the ends of the crura penis; to which he adds a third, less than the other, seated almost in the urethra, a little nearer the glands than the former. All these glands have excretory ducts into the urethra, and from them are secreted all the matter which flows from the urethra in a gonorrhœa, whether venereal or not. In the venereal infection, the urethra and the glands are first inflamed by the contagious matter, that causes a heat of urine, which abates as soon as the glands begin to discharge freely; but if by chance this disease continues till any part of the urethra is ulcerated, the ulcer never heals without a cicatrix, which constricts the urethra, and makes that disease which is vulgarly called a caruncle. The inner texture of the penis is spongy, like the inner texture of the spleen, or the ends of the great bones. It is usually distinguished into corpus cavernosum penis, glandis, and urethræ. The first of these makes part of the glands, and is divided its whole length

length by a ſeptum; the other two are compoſed of ſmaller cells, and are but one body. On the upper ſide of the penis are two arteries, and one vein called vena ipſius penis. The arteries are derived from the beginnings of the umbilical arteries, which parts never dry up, and the vein runs back to the iliac veins. The vena ipſius penis, being obſtructed, the blood that comes by the arteries, diſtends the cells of the whole penis, and makes it erect; but to prevent miſchief from this mechaniſm, there are ſmall collateral veins on the ſurface of the penis, that carry back ſome blood all the time the penis is erect; but by what power the vena ipſius penis is obſtructed to erect the penis, I cannot conceive, unleſs ſmall muſcular fibres conſtrict it. Some think the muſculi erectores penis do it, by thruſting the penis againſt the os pubis; but they ſeem not ſeated conveniently for ſuch an office; beſides, if a preſſure from the lower ſide of the penis is ſufficient, an artificial preſſure, which may be much greater, ſhould, I think, produce the ſame effect.

In the ſeed of men, and of other male animals, Lewenhoeck, by the help of microſcopes, diſcovered an infinite number of animals like tadpoles, which he and others ſuppoſe to be men in miniature, and that one of theſe being entered into an egg in one of the ovaria (ſee the next chapter) conception is performed. But though ſcarce any one, that has made due enquiry, has ever doubted

doubted of the exiſtence of theſe animals, yet there are many who object againſt this hypotheſis; and though I am inclined to think it true, yet I will endeavour impartially to lay down the principal objections and anſwers, that the reader may judge for himſelf. The firſt and ſtrongeſt objection, is raiſed from the ſeveral inſtances that have happened of mixed generation, where the animal produced always appears to partake of both kinds, as in the common caſe of a mule, which is begot by an aſs upon a mare; when, according to that hypotheſis, they expect the animal produced from mixed generation ſhould be entirely of the ſame ſpecies with the male animal; as the ſeeds of plants, whatever earth they grow in, always produce plants of the ſame kind. Neverthleſs, if we conſider what influence womens fears or longings frequently have upon their children in utero, and how great a change caſtration makes in the ſhape of any animal, we cannot then wonder if the mother's blood, to which the animal owes its nouriſhment and increaſe, from the time of impregnation to the time of its birth, ſhould be thought a ſufficient cauſe of reſemblance between theſe animals and their mothers. Another objection is, that nature ſhould provide ſuch a multiplicity of theſe animals, when ſo few can ever be of uſe. To which it has been anſwered, that in plants a very few of the whole that are produced, fall into the earth, and produce plants; and as in plants the

the greateſt part of their ſeeds are the food of animals, ſo the greateſt part of the animalculæ may as well live a time to enjoy their own exiſtence, as any other animal of as low an order. The laſt objection is their ſhape, which, I think, will appear to have no great weight, when we conſider how the eggs of flies produce maggots, which grow up into flies; and the tadpole, produced from the egg of a frog, grows into a form as different from a tadpole as the form of a man: And if theſe animals had produced ſo few at a time, as that their young might have undergone this change in utero, it is highly probable, that we ſhould not ſo much as have ſuſpected theſe analogous changes. But how the animalculæ themſelves are produced, is a difficult queſtion, unleſs by equivocal generation, ſeeing none of them appear to be in a ſtate of encreaſe, but all of a ſize.

In a boy that died of the ſtone, I found a double ureter, each part being dilated to an inch diameter; the pelvis in each kidney to twice its natural bigneſs, and the tubuli urinarii, each as large as the pelvis.

In a man that had never been cut for the ſtone, I found the ureters dilated in ſome places to four inches circumference, and in others but little dilated, and a ſtone that I found in the bladder was leſs than a nutmeg, which muſt have fallen in ſeveral pieces, or both ureters could not have been dilated. From this, and other like obſervations, I think

I think it appears, that the great ſize to which the ureters are uſually extended, in people who are troubled with the ſtone, is owing to ſmall ſtones which ſtick at the entrance into the bladder, until the obſtructed urine, which dilates the ureters, can force them into the bladder.

I HAVE in ſeveral ſubjects found one kidney almoſt conſumed, and once a man with but one kidney; and I have ſeen lymphatics in a diſeaſed teſticle, as large as a crow-quill.

CHAPTER II.

Of the genital parts of women.

THE external parts are the mons veneris, which is that riſing of fat covered with hair above the rima magna upon the os pubis, the great doubling of the ſkin on each ſide the rima called labia, and within theſe a leſſer doubling named nymphæ. Theſe help to cloſe up the orifice of the vagina. The nymphæ are uſually ſaid to ſerve to defend the labia from the urine; but I do not ſee how the labia ſtand more in need of ſuch a defence, than the nymphæ themſelves.

CLITORIS is a ſmall ſpongy, body bearing ſome analogy to the penis in men, but has no urethra. It begins with two crura from the oſſa iſchia, which uniting under the oſſa pubis, it proceeds to the upper part of the nymphæ, where it ends under a ſmall doubling of ſkin, called præputium; and the end which is thus covered is called glans. This is ſaid to be the chief ſeat of pleaſure in coition, in women, as the glans is in men.

A LITTLE lower than this, juſt within the vagina, is the exit of the meatus urinarius.

VAGINA is ſeated between the bladder of urine and the inteſtinum rectum. The texture of it is membranous, and its orifice is contracted with a ſphincter (vid. muſc. ſphincter vaginæ) but the farther part is capacious enough to contain the penis without dilating. Near the beginning of the vagina, immediately behind the orifice of the meatus urinarius, is conſtantly found in children a valve called hymen, which, looking towards the orifice of the vagina, cloſes it; but as children grow up, and the ſphincter vaginæ grows ſtrong enough to contract and cloſe the orifice of the vagina, this valve becoming uſeleſs, ceaſes to encreaſe, and is then known by the name of carunculæ myrtiformes. There have been a few inſtances in which the edges of this growing together, it continued unperforate, until it has been neceſſary to make an inciſion to let out the menſes. The inner part of the vagina is formed into rugæ, which are largeſt in thoſe who have not uſed copulation; and leaſt in thoſe who have had many children. Under theſe rugæ are ſmall glands, whoſe excretory ducts are called lacunæ: Theſe glands ſeparate a mucilaginous matter to lubricate the vagina, eſpecially in coition; and are the ſeat of a gonorrhœa in this ſex, as the glands in the urethra are in the male.

UTERUS is ſeated at the end of the vagina; it is about one inch thick, two broad, and large enough to contain the kernel of a hazel nut; but in women that have had children, a little larger. Its orifice into the vagina is called os tincæ, from the reſemblance it bears to a tench's mouth. It has two round ligaments which go from the ſides of it to the groins through the oblique and tranſverſe muſcles of the abdomen, in the ſame manner as do the ſeminal veſſels in men. This way the gut paſſes in a hernia inteſtinalis in women (vid. muſculi abdominis.) Some authors mention ligamenta lata, which are nothing but a part of the peritonæum. Near the ſides of the uterus lie two bodies called ovaria; they are of a depreſſed oval figure, about half the ſize of men's teſticles, and have ſpermatic veſſels; they contain ſmall pellucid eggs, from which they have their name. There are two arteries and two veins, which paſs to and from the ovaries or teſtes, in the ſame manner that they do in men; but make more windings, and the arteries dilate more ſuddenly, in proportion as they are ſhorter. Theſe arteries and veins detach branches into the uterus and fallopian tubes, and not only make communications betwixt

betwixt the artery and vein on one ſide and thoſe of the other, but alſo with the proper veſſels of the uterus, which are detached from the internal iliac arteries and veins. From theſe veſſels in the inſide of the uterus, the menſtrual purgations are made in women, and ſomething of the ſame kind in brutes, as often as they deſire coition. One uſe of theſe purgations is, to open the veſſels of the uterus, for the veſſels of the placenta to join to them. Many authors have imagined, that there muſt be ſome evacuations analogous to this, in men, which I cannot ſee the neceſſity of; but, on the contrary, I believe that mens not having ſuch evacuations, is the true reaſon why their bodies grows larger and ſtronger than womens: And their continuing to grow longer before they are fit for marriage, I alſo take to be the true reaſon why there are more males born than females, in about the proportion of thirteen to twelve; for women being ſooner fit for marriage than men, fewer will die before that time, than of men.

NEAR the ſides of the ovaria are ſeated the tubæ fallopianæ, one end of which is connected to the uterus, and the ſide to the ovarium by a membrane, the other end is looſe, and being jagged is called morſus diaboli. Among theſe jaggs is a ſmall orifice which leads into the tube, which near this end is about a quarter of an inch diameter, and thence, growing gradually ſmaller, paſſes to the uterus, and enters there with an orifice about the ſize of a hog's briſtle. The uſe of theſe tubes is to convey the male ſeed from the uterus to the ovaria, to impregnate the eggs for conceptions; yet they appear ſo ill adapted to this end, that many have ſuppoſed there muſt be ſome other paſſage from the uterus to the ovaria: But when we conſider the caſe of conceptions found in theſe tubes, and the exact analogy between theſe and the tubes of birds, where we have the moſt undeniable proofs of the ſeed going through the tube, and of the eggs being impregnated that way, and of the eggs coming from the ovarium through the tube, and ſeemingly with much greater difficulty than in women; and beſides, how frequently a matter like the male ſeed (which I ſuppoſe is ſeed) is found in the fallopian tubes of women, as I have found in executed bodies, and in a common whore that died ſuddenly, it appears to me almoſt certain, that the ſeed goes through the fallopian tubes to the ovaria to impregnate eggs, and comes back through the ſame tubes to the uterus. I have ſeen in a woman both the fallopian tubes unperforated, which, upon the foregoing hypotheſis, muſt have cauſed barrenneſs, and ſeed lodged in theſe tubes may have the ſame effect; which I take to be often the caſe of common whores, and women that uſe coition too frequently; and perhaps the fat in the membrane that connects the ovaria to the tubes, may in very fat women ſo keep theſe tubes from the ovaria

as

as to interrupt impregnations; and besides these cases, too much or too little of the menses may destroy or interrupt conceptions; but the latter case, especially in young women, is very rare. From such causes as these, and not from imbecillity, I imagine it is that barrenness oftner proceeds from women than men; and though women do not propagate to so great an age as men, it is not, I believe, for want of being impregnated, but from their menses ceasing, and those vessels being closed which should nourish the fœtus after the impregnation, as if on purpose to prevent the propagation of a feeble and infirm species. And from this consideration, one cannot but think that the perfection of the fœtus, notwithstanding it is first formed in the male seed, depends more upon the female than the male, or else that nature would, for the sake of the species, have been careful to hinder men as well as women from propagating in a declining age.

CHAPTER. III.

Of the fœtus in utero.

THE fœtus in utero is involved in two coats, viz. chorion, which is external, and amnion which immediately incloses the fœtus. They contain a quantity of liquor, which is a proper medium for so tender a being as the fœtus to rest in, and partly secures it from external injuries, as the aqueous humour does the crystalline in the eye; and when the membranes burst at the time of production, this humour lubricates the vagina uteri, to render the birth less difficult. And seeing the stomach of a fœtus in utero is always full of a fluid, like what is contained in the amnion, and the guts not without extrements; we may suppose that this fluid is frequently, during the time of gestation, swallowed by the fœtus, if not for nourishment, at least to keep these parts in use, and to flow through the lacteals, as a quantity of blood from the right ventricle of the heart flows through the lungs before the birth to keep open those passages till the birth, there being after that time no other way of receiving nourishment, and that the fæces found in the guts of a fœtus, are those parts of this fluid that were taken in at the mouth, and were too gross to enter the lacteals. Yet I own it takes off very much from the probability of the opinion of the fœtus's imbibing this liquor,

liquor, that, if I am rightly informed, ſome who have been born with mouths and noſtrils unperforate, have had ſuch fluids and excrements in the inteſtines that other fœtus's have, which muſt be confeſſed, may be derived from the ſalivary glands and from the liver, &c. The following curious paſſage was ſent me by Mr. MONRO. "This liquor contributes nothing to the nouriſhment of "the fœtus, for theſe reaſons; firſt, becauſe, as "you have well obſerved, vaſt numbers of inſtances might be produced, where no paſſage "was to be found for it: I ſhall give you one I "ſaw myſelf in the Hotel de Dieu at Paris in "1718.

"MARY GUERLIN brought fourth two children, "one a complete girl, the other had neither head, "neck, arms, heart, lungs, ſtomach, ſmall guts, "liver, ſpleen, nor pancreas, yet the great guts, "the organs of urine and generation of a female, "and lower extremities were perfect, and of a "natural growth; the umbical vein, after entering "the abdomen, ſplit into a great many branches, "which were diſtributed to the ſeveral parts "in its abdomen. Though it is true that ſoon "after conception, the liquor in the amnion, and "that in the ſtomach of the fœtus reſemble one "another pretty near, yet afterward they differ "exceedingly; for the liquor in the ſtomach is "ſtill gelatinous, thick, and without acrimony, "while the other becomes thinner and more acrid;

"whereas, had the fœtus conſtantly ſwallowed "this liquor, the caſe would have been quite op-"poſite; nay, often it has happened that theſe "waters (as they are commonly called) have been "found quite corrupted, ſtrongly fetid, and ex-"tremely ſharp, while the fœtus, except the in-"juries which the external parts received, was "well and ſound; witneſs the example mentioned "by Bellinger, of a woman who was cured "of a virulent gonorrhœa during her going with "child. And farther, by Malpighius's deline-"ations of the pullus in ovo, it appears to be evi-"dent that the aſitellus ſerves the ſame purpoſe as "the placenta does in viviparous animals, to con-"vey the albumen attenuated by incubation into "the blood-veſſels of the chick, and that none of "the albumen does paſs through the ſaccus colli-"quamenti."

Besides theſe coats, in a cow and many other animals, we find a membrane called alantois; it is incloſed by the chorion together with the amnion, and contains a quantity of water which it receives from the bladder of urine by the urachus. Its uſe ſeems to be to contain the urine, that it might not by the common paſſage be emptied into the liquor of the amnion, of which the fœtus, I am inclined to think, is frequently drinking.

Whether an alantois is to be found with a human fœtus or no, anatomiſts are not agreed, and I cannot give my opinion, having never had a ſufficient

ſufficient opportunity to enquire. But ſurely children having an urachus, one cannot well doubt of an alantois. I have been informed by a gentleman, whoſe probity I can ſufficiently rely on, that he had ſeen a child that had no external genital parts, and made water through the navel. At Henly upon Thames, there is now living a bargeman's child about ten years old, of which I had the like account; but upon examination I found the unperforated glans with its frænum immediately below the place of the navel, and the urine iſſued out by drops between this and the belly, in the place which I ſuppoſe was the navel, but it was ſo much excoriated, that I could make no certain judgment about it. In the uterus of a cow with two calves, I found they had but one chorion, but each an amnion and alantois diſtinct; but the cotyledons, which are analogous to the placenta of the human fœtus, were pretty much in common to the umbilical blood-veſſels of both.

The placenta, or womb-liver, is a maſs of blood-veſſels ſeated on the outſide of the chorion, being compoſed of the extreme branches of the umbilical vein and arteries, which are, for the compoſition of this part, divided into exceeding ſmall branches, to join a like number of the menſtrual veſſels of the uterus; which veſſels of the uterus are made numerous rather than large, that the ſeparation of the placenta from them may not be attended with a flux of blood fatal to the mother;

ther; for the ſides of little veſſels ſoon collapſe and cloſe, and they are more eaſily ſtopped, being compreſſed by the uterus itſelf as it ſhrinks, which it begins to do from the time of the birth; but when the placenta is ſeparated before the delivery, whether untimely or not, theſe veſſels bleed until the uterus is diſcharged of the fœtus. The figure of the placenta is circular, and at its greateſt growth about two inches thick, and ſix or ſeven in diameter.

The arteries and veins of the uterus of the mother, by which the menſtrual purgations are made, are joined to the umbilical arteries and veins in the placenta of the fœtus, the arteries of the uterus to the veins in the placenta, and the veins in the uterus to the arteries of the placenta: By theſe veſſels a large quantity of blood is continually flowing from the mother to the fœtus and back again; but for what end ſuch a quantity flows continually, and back again, I cannot conceive, unleſs it is that the fœtus not breathing for itſelf, it is neceſſary that as much blood of the mother ſhould flow continually to the fœtus, as can leave enough of air, or whatever our blood receives in the lungs, for the fœtus; and perhaps what nutritious juices the fœtus receives, require a great deal of blood to convey them, they being but a ſmall part of the blood. And though the blood paſſes ſo plentifully between the mother and the fœtus, yet the communications are not ſo obvious as they

are

are between the arteries and veins in the ſame body; which makes ſome think the communication is not made by inoſculations of veſſels, but that the fœtus is nouriſhed from the placenta in a vegetable manner; but, I own, I am not of this opinion. The navel-ſtring or umbilical blood-veſſels, between the placenta and the navel, are about two feet long, that the fœtus may have room to move without tearing the placenta from the uterus, which being done too ſoon, from whatever cauſe, occaſions a miſcarriage. Theſe veſſels, viz. two arteries and one vein, twiſt about each other, particularly the arteries about the vein, and are contained in one common coat, together with a veſſel called urachus, which ariſes from the top of the bladder of urine, and ends in the membrana alantois; the umbilical vein goes from the navel directly into the liver, and there enters the great trunk of the vena portæ. Near which entrance, there goes out the ductus venoſus to the great trunk of the cava, which carries part of the blood that is brought by the umbilical vein, that way into the cava, while the reſt circulates with the blood in the porta, the whole of it not paſſing through the ductus venoſus, as is generally believed, but a great part of it into branches of the porta, in the liver, otherwiſe there need be no communication between the umbilical vein and the porta. When the umbilical vein is ſtopped, it becomes a ligament, and the ductus venoſus ſoon ſhrinks and

and almost disappears, having no longer any blood flowing through it; and even the porta itself within the liver, from whence only blood could pass after the birth into the ductus venosus, has less blood flowing through it for some time than it had before the birth, it receiving much blood before the birth from the umbilical vein. The blood which flows from the mother to the fœtus by the umbilical vein, is returned, all but a small quantity, which is reserved for nutrition by the two umbilical arteries, which arise from the internal iliac arteries, and passing by the outsides of the bladder go directly to the navel and placenta; these with the urachus being shrunk up after the birth, lose much of their appearance, especially near the navel, where they are sometimes not to be distinguished.

PART of the blood before the birth, and not the whole quantity, as is generally thought, which is brought by the ascending cava to the right auricle, passes at once through the foramen ovale into the left auricle, and the rest flows into the right ventricle with the blood of the descending cava, and thence into the pulmonary artery, where about one half flows into the lungs, and the other half directly into the aorta by the ductus arteriosus, which lies between the pulmonary artery, and the aorta, which after the birth is called ductus arteriosus in ligamentum versus. The better to explain this contrivance, I will call the quantity of blood

blood flowing through the aſcending cava in a given time, four; and that which flows through the deſcending cava, two: Then let two of the quantity in the aſcending cava flow into the right auricle, it will then with the two received from the deſcending cava have the quantity four; which being thrown from the right ventricle into the pulmonary artery, the quantity two is thrown into the aorta by the ductus arterioſus, and the ſame quantity into the lungs by the pulmonary branches; then the quantity returning from the lungs to the left auricle, will be two in the ſame given time, which being added to the two which flowed through the foramen ovale, in the ſame time there will be conſtantly the ſame proportions received into each ventricle, at every diaſtole of the ventricles, as after the birth. Now if the blood, flowing through the aſcending cava joined by that from the umbilical vein, was but equal to that flowing through the deſcending, let each of them be called two, and let all the blood of the aſcending cava go through the foramen ovale; then the blood which the left ventricle would receive, would exceed that which flows into the right, by the whole quantity which flows from the lungs in the ſame time; but the aſcending cava conveying more blood than the deſcending cava, the exceſs in the left ventricle would be yet greater. If the proportions, which I have taken for the eaſier computing, were perfectly right, as I am ſure they

they are nearly, then the quantity flowing into the left ventricle, would be to that flowing into the right at the ſame time as five to two, if all the aſcending blood went through the foramen ovale.

AND though after the birth the left ventricle of the heart is only employed in throwing blood into the aorta, and the right wholly employed in circulating the blood through the lungs; yet before the birth all the blood thrown out by the left ventricle, and about half the blood thrown out of the right ventricle, being thrown into the aorta, and the other part only through the lungs, it follows, that the whole force exerted by the left ventricle, with about half that of the right, is employed in throwing blood into the aorta, while that diſtributes blood through the whole fœtus and to the mother: But after the birth, when the blood is to be no longer carried from the fœtus to the mother, the left ventricle becomes ſufficient for the circulation through the fœtus, and a new occaſion immediately ariſes for that additional power, which before was neceſſarily employed in throwing blood into the aorta; for the whole maſs of blood now being to be circulated through the lungs, the ductus arterioſus cloſes, and the right ventricle muſt throw all the blood it receives into the lungs, there being no longer any paſſage into the aorta. It is ſuppoſed that the inflation of the lungs at the birth, preſently alters the poſition of the ductus arterioſus, ſo as to obſtruct it; which

 account

account is indeed mechanical, but, I think, not true, becauſe I can neither diſcern that the poſition of this veſſel is altered, nor its ſurface compreſſed: But I rather think that immediately upon the birth, there being no blood carried off from the fœtus to the mother, and the left ventricle being ſufficient to fill the aorta and its branches with blood, as I have ſhewn before, there is no longer room for any blood from the right ventricle; wherefore the blood from the right ventricle will be forced into the lungs, where the paſſage is now made eaſy, as I imagine, by their being inflated; and the ductus arterioſus, having the blood no longer forced into it, ſhrinks, and in time almoſt diſappears. This duct being ſtopped, the valve of the foramen ovale ſoon ſtops that paſſage, it being on the ſide of the left auricle (or that muſcular bag, which is the largeſt part of that auricle) which being much the ſtrongeſt, the valve muſt be preſſed more on that ſide than the other, by the blood, in the time of the ſyſtole of the auricle; and it is as evident, that in the diaſtole of the auricle, there muſt be more preſſure to open that than the right, it being a ſtronger muſcle, or elſe there could have been no reaſon for having the left auricle ſtronger than the right, in proportion to their ventricles. Sometimes this valve does not quite cover the foramen, in which caſe a ſmall quantity of blood may poſſibly flow from the left auricle to the right, and ſo circulate

twice

twice through the lungs to once through the body, but none could flow from the right to the left and eſcape the lungs, which might be of bad conſequence. Some have imagined, that men, who have this paſſage open, cannot be drowned: But though this paſſage is ſometimes found open, no man has been yet ſeen, that we have ever heard of, that could not be drowned. I have ſeen the foramen open in a man that was hanged, to whom one might juſtly expect it ſhould have been as uſeful as in the caſe of ſubmerſion in water. Many writers have ſuppoſed, that this foramen is open in amphibious animals, and in ſuch fiſhes as have two auricles, two ventricles, and lungs like land animals, without gills, which in other fiſh are analogous to lungs. I have diſſected a porpoiſe, which is of this kind, and found this foramen cloſed; but the great veins were vaſtly large in proportion to the bulk of the animal; whence I conjectured, their blood was accumulated in their veins, while they kept under water, and by that means the lungs eſcaped being oppreſſed with blood; which conjecture ſeemed to me the more probable, ſince all animals of this kind are able to abide the leaſt time under water, when their blood is moſt expanded with heat. But upon the diſſection of an otter, whoſe foramen ovale was alſo cloſed, I found the veins nothing differing from thoſe of other animals. In a water-tortoiſe, which I had an opportunity of examining, with that

moſt

most dextrous and indefatigable anatomist Dr. DOUGLASS, I found the two ventricles of the heart but half divided by a septum, and in the beginning of the pulmonary artery several strong muscular rings, a little distance from each other, each of which by contracting, would be capable of resisting a part of that blood, which otherwise would have been thrown into the lungs, when they were under water; and this blood so obstructed must necessarily be thrown into the aorta, the two ventricles being in a manner one common cavity; and when they are out of the water, this communication of ventricles will suffer but little confusion of the blood which flows into the ventricles, because each ventricle receiving and discharging the same quantity of blood, at the same time, they will balance each other, and thereby such a mixture will be very much prevented. Mr. MONRO observes, that the water-tortoise has very large lungs, consisting of larger vesicles than land animals, and that they receive a greater quantity of air to furnish that je ne sçai quoi so necessary for the life of animals: The same thing I have observed in frogs.

As to the reason of womens bringing forth at the usual time; it has been said, that at that time, the head of the child begins to be specifically heavier than the rest of the body, and therefore must fall lowest in the fluid it lies in, which being an uneasy posture, makes the child struggle, and bring on the labour. But it is not true, that the head then alters its ſpecific gravity; or, if it did, there is ſeldom fluid enough in the amnion for this purpoſe; and beſides, this could only happen right in one poſture, and would uſually happen wrong in brutes.

CHAPTER IV.

Of the eye.

THE figure, ſituation, and uſe of the eyes, together with the eye-brows, eye-laſhes, and eye-lids, being well known, I need only deſcribe what is uſually ſhewn by diſſecting. The orbit of the eye, or cavity in which it is contained, is in all the vacant places filled with a looſe fat, which is a proper medium for the eye to reſt in, and ſerves as a ſocket for it to be moved in. In the upper and outer part of the orbit, is ſeated the lacrymal gland. Its uſe is to furniſh at all times water enough to waſh off duſt, and to keep the outer ſurface of the eye moiſt, without which the tunica cornea would be leſs pellucid, and the rays of light would be diſturbed in their paſſage; and that this liquor may be rightly diſpoſed of, we frequently cloſe the eye-lids to ſpread it equally, even when we are not conſcious of doing it. At the inner corner of the eye, between the eye-lids,

ſtands

ſtands a caruncle, which ſeems to be placed to keep that corner of the eye-lids from being totally cloſed, that any tears or gummy matter may flow from under the eye-lids, when we ſleep, or into the puncta lacrymalia, which are little holes, one in each eye-lid, near this corner, to carry off into the ductus ad naſum, any ſuperfluous tears.

THE firſt membrane of the eye is called conjunctiva; it covers ſo much of the eye as is called the white, and being reflected all round, it lines the two eye-lids; it being thus returned from the eye to the inſide of the eye-lids, it effectually hinders any extraneous bodies from getting behind the eye into the orbit, and ſmooths the parts it covers, which makes the friction leſs between the eye and the eye-lids. This coat is very full of blood-veſſels, as appears upon any inflammation.

TUNICA SCLEROTIS, and CORNEA, make together one firm caſe of a proper form, for the uſe of the other coats and humours. The fore part of this ſtrong coat being tranſparent, and like horn, is called cornea, and the reſt ſclerotis. Under the cornea lies the iris, which is an opake membrane, like the tunica choroides, but of different colours in different eyes, ſuch as the eye appears, as grey, black, or hazel; for being ſeated under the tunica cornea, it gives ſuch an appearance to that as it has itſelf. The middle of it is perforated for the admiſſion of the rays of light, and is called the pupil. Immediately under the

the iris lie the processus ciliares, like radial lines from a lesser circle to a greater. When these processes contract, they dilate the pupil to suffer more rays of light to enter into the eye; and the contrary is done by the circular fibres of the iris, which act as a sphincter muscle: But these changes are not made with great quickness, as appears from the eyes being oppressed with a strong light for some time, after we come out of a dark place, and from the contrary effect in going suddenly from a light place to a dark one. And as the pupil always dilates in darker places, to receive more rays of light, so when any disease makes some of those rays ineffectual, which pass through the pupil, it dilates as in dark places to admit more light; therefore a dilated pupil is a certain sign of a bad eye, and this may be discerned usually sooner than the patient discerns any defect in vision. In men the pupil is round, which fits them to see every way alike; it is also round in animals that are the prey both of birds and beasts. But graminivorous brutes, that are too large to be the prey of birds, have it oblong horizontally, which fits them to view a large space upon the earth; while animals of the cat kind, who climb trees and prey indifferently on birds or animals that hide in the earth, have their pupils oblong the contrary way, which fits them best to look upward and downward at once. Besides these there are other animals whose pupils are in these forms, but in less proportions,

proportions, ſo as beſt to fit their ways of life. Immediately under the ſclerotis, is a membrane of little firmneſs, called choroides. In men it is of a ruſty dark colour, ſuch as will bury almoſt all the rays of light, that paſs through the tunica retina, which if it were of a brighter colour, would reflect many of the rays upon the retina, and make a ſecond image upon the firſt ſomewhat leſs, and leſs diſtinct, but both together ſtronger; which is the caſe of brutes of prey, where a great part of this coat is perfectly white, which makes them ſee bodies of all colours in the night better than men, for white reflects all colours: But brutes that feed only on graſs, have the ſame parts of this membrane of a bright green, which enables them alſo to ſee with leſs light, and makes graſs an object that they can diſcern with greateſt ſtrength. But theſe advantages in brutes neceſſarily deſtroy great accuracy in viſion, which is of little or no uſe to them, but to men of great conſequence. This green part of the tunica choroides in animals that graze, may properly be called membrana uvea, from its reſemblance in colour to an unripe grape. But in mens eyes only a white circle round the back ſide of the choroides near the cornea, is called uvea.

Immediately under the tunica choroides, lies the tunica retina, which is the optic nerve expanded and co-extended with the choroides. Rays of light ſtriking upon this membrane, the

 ſenſation

ſenſation is conveyed by the optic nerves, to the common ſenſorium the brain; theſe nerves do not enter at the middle of the bottom of the eyes, but nearer the noſe; for thoſe rays of light being ineffectual for viſion that fall upon the entrance of the optic nerves, it is fit they ſhould ſo enter, as that the ſame object, or part of any object, ſhould not be unperceived in both eyes, as would have been the caſe, had they been otherwiſe inſerted; which appears from a common experiment of part of an object being loſt to one eye, when we are looking towards it with the other ſhut. I know a gentleman, who having loſt one eye by the ſmall-pox, and going through a hedge, a thorn unſeen (probably from this cauſe) ſtruck the other and put it out. The two optic nerves, ſoon after they ariſe out of the brain, join, and ſeem perfectly united; yet from the following caſe I am not without ſuſpicion of their fibres being preſerved diſtinct, and that the nerve of each eye ariſes wholly from the oppoſite ſide of the brain, or elſe that the other nerves throughout the body ariſe from the brain, and medulla oblongata, on the ſides oppoſite to thoſe they come out of. A ſoldier, who was my patient in the hoſpital about five years ſince, had, by a puſh with a broad ſword, his left eye raiſed in the orbit, which I replaced with my fingers; it was preſently followed with exceſſive pain in the right ſide of the head only; and a loſs of the ſenſe of feeling and motion

motion in both the right limbs; the ſenſe of feeling he recovered by degrees in about a month, and ſoon after began to recover their motion, but was twelve months before he could walk, and lift up his hand to his head; and in about two years recovered all but the ſight of the wounded eye, which indeed did not appear perfect. In fiſh theſe nerves ariſe diſtinct from the oppoſite ſides of the brain, and croſs without uniting; but as theſe animals have their eyes ſo placed, as not to ſee the ſame object with both eyes at once, whereas animals, whoſe optic nerves ſeem to unite, do ſee the ſame object with both eyes at once, one would ſuſpect that in one they were joined to make the object not appear double, and in the other diſtinct, to make their two eyes (as they are to view different objects at the ſame time) independent on each other: And yet from the following caſes, the ſeeing objects ſingle ſeems not to depend upon any ſuch union, nor from the light ſtriking upon correſponding fibres of the nerves, as others have believed, but upon a judgment from experience, all objects appearing ſingle to both eyes in the manner we are moſt uſed to obſerve them, but in other caſes double; for though we have a diſtinct image from each eye ſent to the brain, yet while both theſe images are of an object ſeen in one and the ſame place, we conceive of them as one; ſo when one image appears to the eyes (when they are diſtorted or wrong directed) in two different places, it gives the idea of two; and when two bodies are seen in one place, as two candles rightly placed, through one hole in a board, they appear one. But cases of this kind being too numerous, I will conclude with one very remarkable, and, I think, much in favour of this opinion. A gentleman, who from a blow on the head, had one eye distorted, found every object appear double, but by degrees the most familiar ones became single, and in time, all objects became so, without any amendment of the distortion.

The inside of the eye is filled with three humours, called aqueous, crystalline, and vitreous. The aqueous lies foremost, and seems chiefly of use to prevent the crystalline from being easily bruised by rubbing, or a blow; and perhaps it serves for the crystalline humour to move forward in, while we view near objects, and backward for remoter objects; without which mechanism, or, in the place of it, a greater convexity in the crystalline humour in the former case, and a less convexity in the latter, I do not imagine, according to the laws of optics, how we could so distinctly see objects at different distances. However it is in land-animals, I think, we may plainly see, that fish move their crystalline humour nearer the bottom of the eye when they are out of water, and the contrary way in water; because light is less refracted from water through the crystalline humour

mour than from air. Some have ſaid, that amphibious animals have a membrane like the membrana nictitans of birds, which ſerves them as a lens in the water. I have examined the eye of a crocodile, which Sir HANS SLOAN kept in ſpirits, and I found this membrane equally thick and denſe, and conſequently unfit for this purpoſe, or, I believe, any other, except that obvious one, of defending the eye from the water. Next behind the aqueous humour lies the cryſtalline; its ſhape is a depreſſed ſpheroid, it is diſtinctly contained in a very fine membrane called aranea. The uſe of this humour is to refract the rays of light which paſs through it, ſo that each pencil of rays from the ſame point of any object, may be united upon the retina, as in a camera obſcura, to make the ſtronger impreſſion; and though by this union of the rays, a picture inverted is made upon the retina, yet ſurely it is the impulſe only of the rays upon the retina, that is the cauſe of viſion; for had the colour of the retina been black, and conſequently unfit to receive ſuch a picture, would not the impulſe of light upon it have been ſufficient for viſion? or would ſuch a picture, if it could have been made without any impulſe, have ever conveyed any ſenſation to the brain? Then if the impulſe of light upon the retina, and not the image upon the retina, is the cauſe of viſion; when we enquire why an image inverted in the eye appears otherwiſe to the mind, might we we not expect to find the true cauſe from conſidering the directions in which the rays ſtrike the retina, as we judge of above and below from a like experience, when any thing ſtrikes upon any part of our bodies? Nevertheleſs, in viewing an object through a lens, we conceive of it as inverted; whenas in receiving the impulſes of light in the ſame manner, and having the picture on the retina in the ſame attitude, when we ſtand on our heads without the lens, we have not the ſame, but the contrary idea of the poſition of the object. Though I have conſidered this humour only as a refractor of light, yet the firſt and greateſt refraction is undoubtedly made in the cornea; but it being concavo-convex, like glaſſes of that kind, while one ſide makes the rays of light converge, the other diverges them again. The ſame thing alſo may be obſerved of the aqueous humour, which is indeed more concave than convex; but when the cryſtalline humour is removed in the couching a cataract, the aqueous poſſeſſes its place and becomes a lens; but that refracting light leſs than the cryſtalline, whoſe place and ſhape it partly takes, the patient needs a convex glaſs to ſee accurately. In ſome eyes, either this humour being too convex or too diſtant from the retina, the rays unite too ſoon, unleſs the object is held very near to the eye, which fault is remediable by a concave glaſs; as the contrary fault, common to old perſons, is by a convex glaſs. If the eye

had

had been formed for a nearer view, the object would often obſtruct the light; if it had been much farther, light enough would not commonly have been produced from the object to the eye. In fiſh the cryſtalline humour ſeems a perfect ſphere, which is neceſſary for them, becauſe light being leſs refracted from water through the cryſtalline humour than from air, that defect is compenſated by a more convex lens. The vitreous humour lies behind the cryſtalline, and fills up the greateſt part of the eye: Its fore ſide is concave for the cryſtalline humour to lodge in, and its back ſide being convex, the tunica retina is ſpread over it; it ſerves as a medium to keep the cryſtalline humour and the retina at a due diſtance.

THE larger animals having larger eyes, their organs of viſion, like a microſcope with a large lens, are fit to take in a greater view, but in that view things are not ſo much magnified; in leſſer animals a ſmall ſpace is diſcerned, ſuch as is their ſphere of action, but that greatly magnified, not really ſo in either caſe, but comparatively, for viſion ſhews not the real magnitude of objects, but their proportions one to another. Fiſh have their eyes, and particularly their pupils, larger than land animals, becauſe there is leſs light, and that not ſo far diſtributed in water as in the air. In all inflammations in the eye, the utmoſt haſte ſhould be made by bleeding, purging, abſtinence, &c. to get rid of the inflammation, becauſe a continued

tinued inflammation ſeldom fails to make white opake ſcars in the cornea, which cauſe dimneſs if not blindneſs; and no eye-water with powders in it ſhould ever be put upon the eye, becauſe none can be made fine enough.

An account of obſervations made by a young gentleman who was born blind, or loſt his ſight ſo early that he had no remembrance of ever having ſeen, and was couched between thirteen and fourteen years of age.

THO' we ſay of this gentleman that he was blind, as we do of all people who have ripe cataracts, yet they are never ſo blind from that cauſe but that they can diſcern day from night, and for the moſt part, in a ſtrong light, diſtinguiſh black, white, and ſcarlet; but they cannot perceive the ſhape of any thing; for the light by which theſe perceptions are made, being let in obliquely through the aqueous humour, or the anterior ſurface of the cryſtalline, by which the rays cannot be brought into a focus upon the retina, they can diſcern in no other manner, than a ſound eye can through a glaſs of broken jelly, where a great variety of ſurfaces ſo differently refract the light, that the ſeveral diſtinct pencils of rays cannot be collected by the eye into their proper foci; wherefore the ſhape of an object in ſuch a caſe cannot be at all diſcerned, though the colour may:

And thus it was with this young gentleman, who though he knew theſe colours aſunder in a good light, yet when he ſaw them after he was couched, the faint ideas he had of them before, were not ſufficient for him to know them by afterwards, and therefore he did not think them the ſame which he had before known by thoſe names. Now ſcarlet he thought the moſt beautiful of all colours, and of others the moſt gay were the moſt pleaſing; whereas the firſt time he ſaw black it gave him great uneaſineſs, yet after a little time he was reconciled to it; but ſome months after, ſeeing by accident a negro woman, he was ſtruck with great horror at the ſight.

WHEN he firſt ſaw, he was ſo far from making any judgment about diſtances, that he thought all objects whatever touched his eyes (as he expreſſed it) as what he felt did his ſkin, and thought no objects ſo agreeable as thoſe which were ſmooth and regular, though he could form no judgment of their ſhape, or gueſs what it was in any object that was pleaſing to him: He knew not the ſhape of any thing, nor any one thing from another, however different in ſhape or magnitude; but upon being told what things were, whoſe form he before knew from feeling, he would carefully obſerve, that he might know them again; but having too many objects to learn at once, he forgot many of them; and (as he ſaid) at firſt he learned to know, and again forgot a thouſand things

things in a day. One particular only, though it may appear trifling, I will relate: Having often forgot which was the cat, and which the dog, he was aſhamed to aſk; but catching the cat, which he knew by feeling, he was obſerved to look at her ſtedfaſtly, and then, ſetting her down, ſaid, So puſs, I ſhall know you another time. He was very much ſurprized, that thoſe things which he had liked beſt, did not appear moſt agreeable to his eyes, expecting thoſe perſons would appear moſt beautiful that he loved moſt, and ſuch things to be moſt agreeable to his ſight, that were ſo to his taſte. We thought he ſoon knew what pictures repreſented, which were ſhewed to him, but we found afterwards we were miſtaken; for about two months after he was couched, he diſcovered at once they repreſented ſolid bodies, when to that time he conſidered them only as party coloured planes, or ſurfaces diverſified with variety of paint; but even then he was no leſs ſurprized, expecting the pictures would feel like the things they repreſented, and was amazed when he found thoſe parts, which by their light and ſhadow appeared now round and uneven, felt only flat like the reſt, and aſked which was the lying ſenſe, feeling, or ſeeing?

Being ſhewn his father's picture in a locket at his mother's watch, and told what it was, he acknowledged a likeneſs, but was vaſtly ſurprized; aſking, how it could be, that a large face could be expreſſed in ſo little room, ſaying, it ſhould have ſeemed as impoſſible to him, as to put a buſhel of any thing into a pint.

At firſt, he could bear but very little ſight, and the things he ſaw, he thought extremely large; but upon ſeeing things larger, thoſe firſt ſeen he conceived leſs, never being able to imagine any lines beyond the bounds he ſaw; the room he was in, he ſaid, he knew to be but part of the houſe, yet he could not conceive that the whole houſe could look bigger. Before he was couched, he expected little advantage from ſeeing, worth undergoing an operation for, except reading and writing; for he ſaid, he thought he could have no more pleaſure in walking abroad than he had in the garden, which he could do ſafely and readily. And even blindneſs, he obſerved, had this advantage, that he could go any where in the dark, much better than thoſe who can ſee; and after he had ſeen, he did not ſoon loſe this quality, nor deſire a light to go about the houſe in the night. He ſaid, every new object was a new delight; and the pleaſure was ſo great, that he wanted words to expreſs it; but his gratitude to his operator he could not conceal, never ſeeing him for ſome time without tears of joy in his eyes, and other marks of affection: And if he did not happen to come at any time when he was expected, he would be ſo grieved, that he could not forbear crying at his diſappointment. A year after firſt ſeeing, being carried

carried upon Epſom Downs, and obſerving a large proſpect, he was exceedingly delighted with it, and called it a new kind of ſeeing. And now, being lately couched of his other eye, he ſays, that objects at firſt appeared large to this eye, but not ſo large as they did at firſt to the other; and looking upon the ſame object with both eyes, he thought it looked about twice as large as with the firſt couched eye only, but not double, that we can any ways diſcover.

I HAVE couched ſeveral others who were born blind, whoſe obſervations were of the ſame kind; but they being younger, none of them gave ſo full an account as this gentleman.

CHAPTER V.

Of the ear.

THE figure and ſituation of the outer ear needs no deſcription: Its inner ſubſtance is cartilage, which preſerves its form without being liable to break: Its uſe is to collect ſounds, and direct them into the meatus auditorius, which is the paſſage that leads to the drum; this paſſage is lined with a glandular membrane, in which alſo is ſome hair; the cerumen which is ſeparated by theſe glands, being ſpread all over this membrane, and its hairs, ſerve to defend the membrane from the outer

outer air, and to entangle any inſect that might otherwiſe get into the ear. Sometimes this wax being ſeparated in too great quantity, it fills up the paſſage and cauſes deafneſs; and thoſe great diſcharges of matter from the meatus auditorius, which are commonly called impoſthumes in the ear, I think, can be nothing elſe than ulcerations, or great ſecretions from theſe glands. At the farther end of the meatus auditorius lies the membrana tympani, which is extended upon a bony ridge almoſt circular: Its ſituation in men and brutes is nearly horizontal, inclined towards the meatus auditorius, which is the beſt poſition to receive ſounds; a great part of them being ordinarily reverberated from the earth. In men and brutes it is concave outward, but in birds it is convex outward, ſo as to make the upper ſide of it nearly perpendicular to the horizon, which ſeems fitter to hear each other's ſounds when they are high in the air, where they can receive but little reverberated ſound. This membrane does not entirely cloſe the paſſage, but has on one ſide a ſmall aperture covered with a valve. I found it once half open in a man that I diſſected, who had not been deaf; and I have ſeen a man ſmoak a whole pipe of tobacco out through his ears, which muſt go from the mouth through the euſtachian tube, and through the tympanum; yet this man heard perfectly well. Theſe caſes occaſioned me to break the tympanum in both ears of a dog, and it did not deſtroy his hearing, but for

 ſome

ſome time he received ſtrong ſounds with great horror. Mr. St. Andre has aſſured me, that a patient of his had the tympanum deſtroyed by an ulcer, and the auditory bones caſt out, without deſtroying his hearing. From theſe, and other like caſes, it may be concluded, that the membrana tympani, though uſeful in hearing, is not the ſeat of that ſenſe; and if any diſeaſe in that membrane ſhould obſtruct the paſſage of ſounds to the internal parts of the ear, which are the ſeat of that ſenſe, an artificial paſſage through that membrane might recover hearing, as the removing the cryſtalline humour, when that obſtructs the light, recovers ſight. Some years ſince a malefactor was pardoned on condition that he ſuffered this experiment, but he falling ill of a fever the operation was deferred, during which time there was ſo great a public clamor raiſed againſt it that it was afterwards thought fit to be forbid. In very young children I have always found this membrane covered with mucus, which ſeems neceſſary to prevent ſounds from affecting them too much, there being no proviſion to ſhut the ears, as there is for the eyes. A gentleman well known in this city, having had four children born deaf, was adviſed to lay bliſters upon the heads of the next children he might have, which he did to three which were born afterward, and every one of them heard well. It ſeems not unreaſonable to ſuppoſe that too great a quantity of this mucus upon the drum might be the cauſe of deafneſs in the four children, and that the diſcharge made by the bliſters in the latter caſes was the cauſe of their eſcaping the ſame misfortune.

INTO the middle of the tympanum is extended a ſmall bone called malleus, whoſe other end is articulated to a bone called incus, which is alſo articulated by the intervention of an exceeding ſmall one, called orbiculare, to a fourth bone called ſtapes. Theſe bones are contained in that cavity behind the tympanum, which is called the barrel of the ear; but ſome anatomiſts call the barrel only tympanum, and the membrane membrana tympani. The malleus being moved inward by the muſculus obliquus internus, or trochlearis, it extends the tympanum that it may be the more affected by impulſe of ſounds when they are too weak. This muſcle ariſes from the cartilaginous part of the euſtachian tube, and paſſing from thence in a proper groove, it is reflected under a ſmall proceſs, and thence paſſes on perpendicular to the tympanum, to be inſerted into the handle of the malleus, ſometimes with a double tendon. Parallel to this muſcle lies another extenſor of the tympanum, called obliquus externus; it ariſes from the outer and upper part of the euſtachian tube, and paſſing through the ſame hole with the corda tympani, which is a branch of the fifth pair of nerves, it is inſerted into a long proceſs of the malleus: This is not ſo obviouſly an extenſor as to be known to be ſo without an experiment. The muſcle which relaxes this membrane is called externus tympani; it arises from the upper part of the auditory passage, under the membrane which lines that passage, and is inserted into the upper process of the malleus. The relaxation of the tympanum is made by this muscle, without our knowledge, when sounds are too strong; and as the pupil of the eye is contracted when we have too much light, and dilated where there is too little, from what cause soever, so when sounds are too low, or the sense of hearing imperfect, from whatever cause, the extensors of the tympanum stretch it to make the impulse of sounds more effectual upon it, just as in the case of the common drum, and the cords of any musical instrument. From the cavity behind the tympanum, which is called the barrel of the ear, goes the eustachian tube, or iter ad palatum; it ends cartilaginous behind the palate. This passage seems to be exactly of the same use with the hole in the side of the common drum, that is, to let the air pass in and out from the barrel of the ear to make the membrane vibrate the better, and perhaps in the ear, which is closer than a common drum, to let air in or out as it alters in density; and if any fluid should be separated in the barrel of the ear, to give it a passage out. This passage being obstructed, as it is sometimes, by a large polypus behind the uvula, it causes great difficulty of hearing, and sometimes, when the meatus auditorius is obstructed, a man opening his mouth wide, will hear pretty well through this paſſage, which is often ſo open, as that ſyringing water through the noſe, it ſhall paſs through into the barrel of the ear, and cauſe deafneſs for ſome time. If any one would try how he can hear this way, let him ſtop his ears, and take between his teeth the end of a wire, or cord that will vibrate well, and holding the other end, ſtrike it, and the ſound that he hears will be through this paſſage. To the ſtapes there is one muſcle called muſculus ſtapedis; it lies in a long channel, and ending in the ſtapes, it ſerves to pull the ſtapes off of the feneſtra ovalis, which otherwiſe it covers. Beſides the feneſtra ovalis, there is another near it ſomewhat leſs, called rotunda; theſe two holes lead to a cavity called veſtibulum, which leads into other cavities aptly called cochlea, and three ſemicircular canals, or altogether the labyrinth, in which are ſpread the auditory nerves, to receive, and convey the impulſe of ſounds to the common ſenſorium the brain; and ſurely the chorda tympani, which is a branch of the fifth pair of nerves, may alſo convey theſe ſenſations to the brain. The two holes, called feneſtra ovalis & rotunda, are cloſed with a fine membrane, like the membrane called the drum, and the larger being occaſionally covered and uncovered by the ſtapes, ſounds are thereby made to influence more or leſs, as beſt ſerves for hearing; and this advantage being added to that of a lax or tenſe tympanum, the effect of ſounds may be greatly encreaſed or leſſened upon the auditory nerves, expanded in the labyrinth. In the ſtrongeſt ſounds, the tympanum may be lax, and the feneſtra ovalis covered; and for the loweſt, the tympanum tenſe and the feneſtra uncovered. If ſounds propagated in the air were heard leſs, we might often be in danger before we were apprized of it; and if the organs of hearing were much more perfect, unleſs our underſtandings were ſo too, we ſhould commonly hear more things at once than we could attend to.

CHAPTER VI.

Of the ſenſes of ſmelling, taſting, and feeling.

THE ſenſe of ſmelling is made by the effluvia, which are conveyed by the air to the nerves, ending in the membranes which line the noſe and its lamellæ. In men theſe lamellæ are few, and the paſſage through the noſe not difficult; hence fewer effluvia will ſtrike the nerves, than in animals of more exquiſite ſmell, whoſe noſes being full of lamellæ, and the paſſage for the air narow and crooked, few of the effluvia eſcape one place or another; beſides, their olfactory nerves may be more ſenſible. Fiſh, though they have no noſes, yet in their mouths they may taſte effluvia in the water, as ſurely thoſe fiſh do, who ſeek their prey in in the darkeſt nights, and in great depths of water, there being more nerves diſpoſed in their mouths, than through their whole bodies beſide, the optic excepted; and it ſeems as if it was done for this purpoſe; for the mere ſenſe of taſting is ordinarily leſs curious in them, than in land animals; in baiting eel-baſkets, if the bait has lain long in water, it is ſeldom followed; but upon ſcarifying it afreſh, which will make it emit new effluvia, it ſerves as a freſh bait. The ſenſe of taſting is made in the like manner upon the nerves which line the mouth, as is that of feeling upon the nerves diſtributed throughout the body; of which I ſhould ſpeak more in this place, if I had not done it already in the chapter of the nerves.

TAB. XXXI.

1 The under ſide of the bladder.
2 The ureters.
3 Vaſa deferentia.
4 Veſiculæ ſeminales.
5 The proſtate gland.
6 Meatus urinarius.
7 A tranſverſe ſection of the corpora cavernoſa penis.
8 Corpus cavernoſum urethræ.
9 Urethra.
10 Septum penis.
11 The ſeptum between the corpus cavernoſum urethræ, and that of the penis.
12 The corpora cavernoſa penis divided by the ſeptum.
13 Corpus cavernoſum glandis.

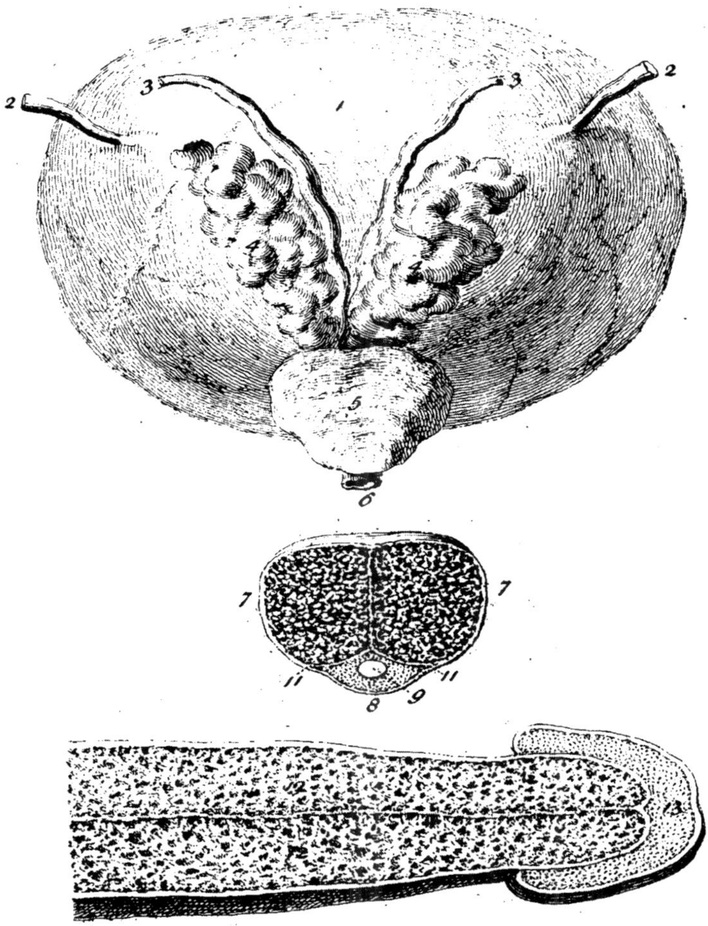
1
2
2
3
3
4
4
5
6
7
7
11
11
8
9
12
13

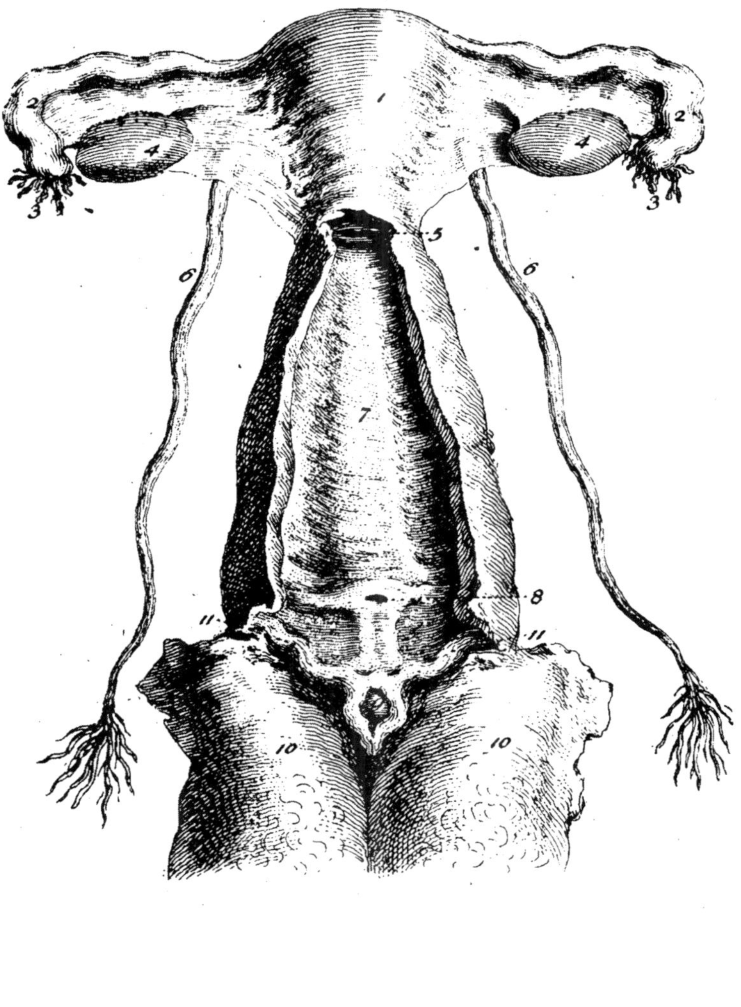
1
2
2
3
3
4
4
5
6
6
7
8
10
10
11
11

TAB. XXXII.

1 That side of the uterus which is next the gut.
2 The fallopian tubes.
3 The fimbriæ.
4 Ovaria.
5 The mouth of the uterus.
6 Ligamenta rotunda,
7 The inside of the vagina.
8 The orifice of the meatus urinarius.
9 The glans clitoridis.
10 The external labia of the vagina.
11 The nymphæ, which are continued from the præputium clitoridis.

TAB. XXXIII.

TAB. XXXIII.

THE parts of an hermaphrodite negro, which was neither ſex perfect, but a wonderful mixture of both. This perſon was twenty-ſix years of age, and in ſhape perfectly male.

1 A clitoris, when erected, almoſt as large as a penis.

2 The glans of the clitoris.

3 Labia, or a divided ſcrotum; in which were perfect teſticles with all the veſſels.

4 Nymphæ.

5 The entrance into the vagina, where were carunculæ myrtiformes.

6 Furca virginis.

THE lower figure repreſents another hermaphrodite, whoſe ſhape was rather female than male, but too young to have female breaſts, or a beard, like a male, upon the face.

7 The glans clitoridis.

8 Nymphæ.

9 Labia with teſticles in them, divaricated to ſhew the parts between, but in their natural ſituation very like the other, as the other when divaricated reſembled this.

10 The entrance into the vagina.

11 Furca virginis.

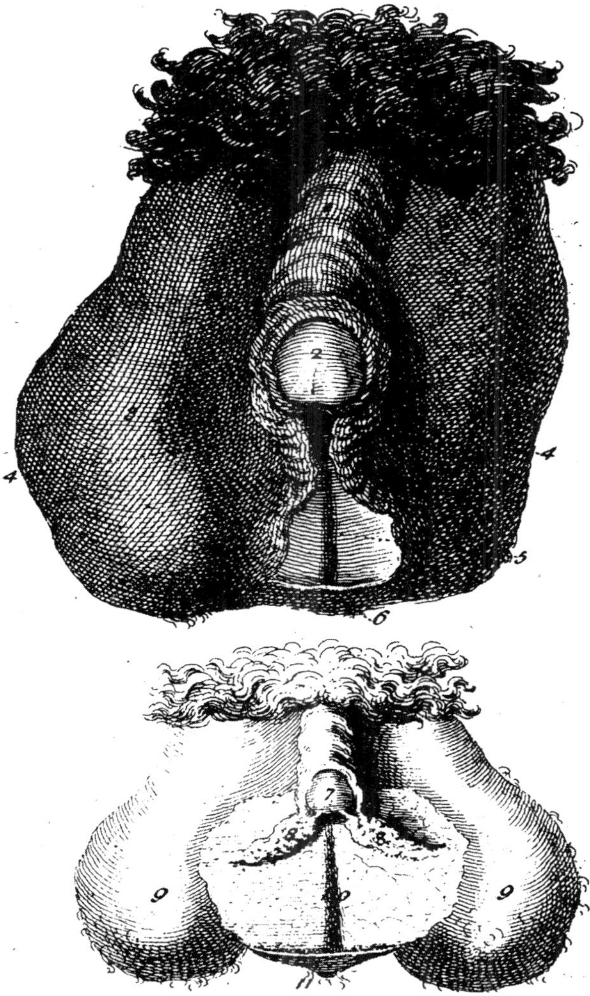
2
4
4
5
6
7
8
8
9
9
11

TAB. XXXIV.

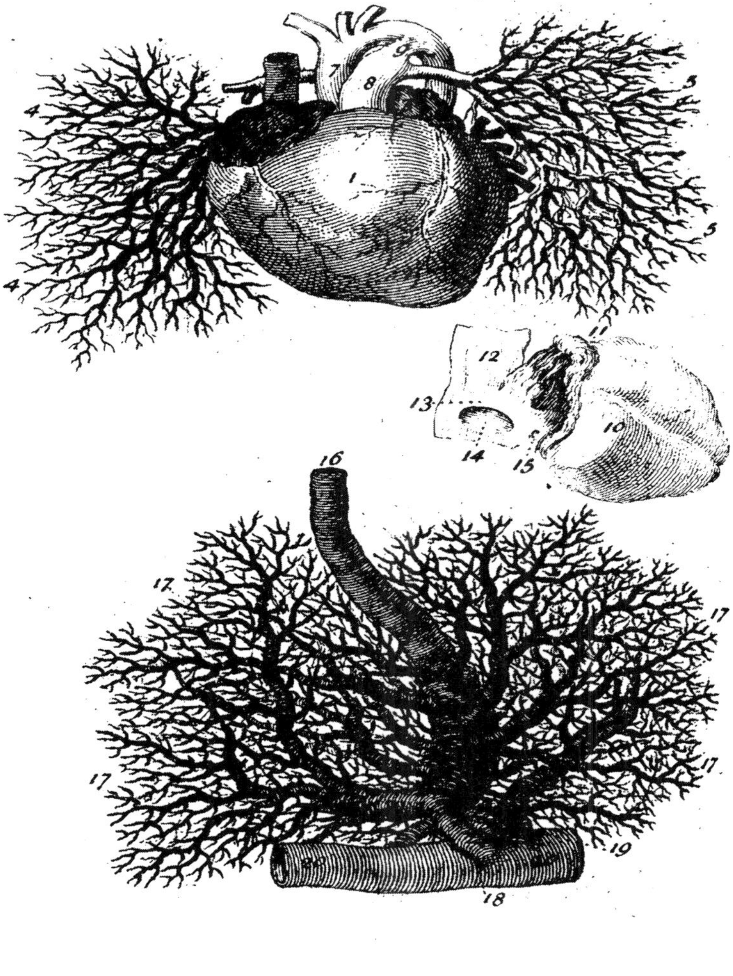

TAB. XXXIV.

1 The right ventricle of a fœtus diſtended with wax.
2 The right auricle.
3 The left auricle.
4 Branches of the pulmonary veins of the right lobe of the lungs, thoſe of the left being cut off ſhort.
5 The arteries of the left lobe of the lungs.
6 The vena cava deſcendens.
7 Aorta aſcendens.
8 Arteria pulmonalis.
9 Ductus arterioſus.
10 The under ſide of a heart of a younger fœtus.
11 The right auricle cut open.
12 The cava deſcendens cut open.
13 Tuberculum loweri.
14 The foramen ovale cloſed with its valve.
15 The mouth of the coronary veins.
16 The umbilical vein.
17 Branches of the vena porta in the liver.
18 Ductus venoſus.
19 Branches of the cava in the liver.
20 Vena cava.

TAB. XXXV.

1 A crofs for an object.
2 The object reprefented on the retina at the bottom of each eye.
3 The entrance of the optic nerves, in which place no object is reprefented.
4 Cones, within which all objects placed are dark to each eye, the rays from thence falling upon the entrance of the optic nerves; but that which falls upon the entrance of the optic nerve in one eye, can never fall upon the optic nerve in the other.
5 Pencils of rays from points of the object paffing through the cryftalline humour, where they converge, to meet in a point on the retina to form vifion.

TAB. XXXVI.

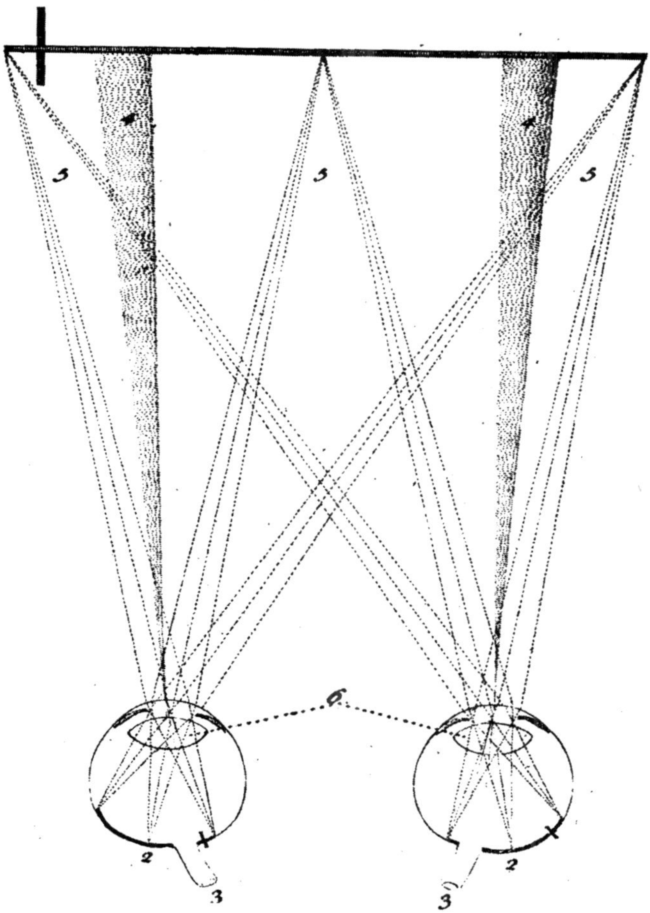
5
5
5
6
2
3
2
3

TAB.XXXVI.

p. 317.

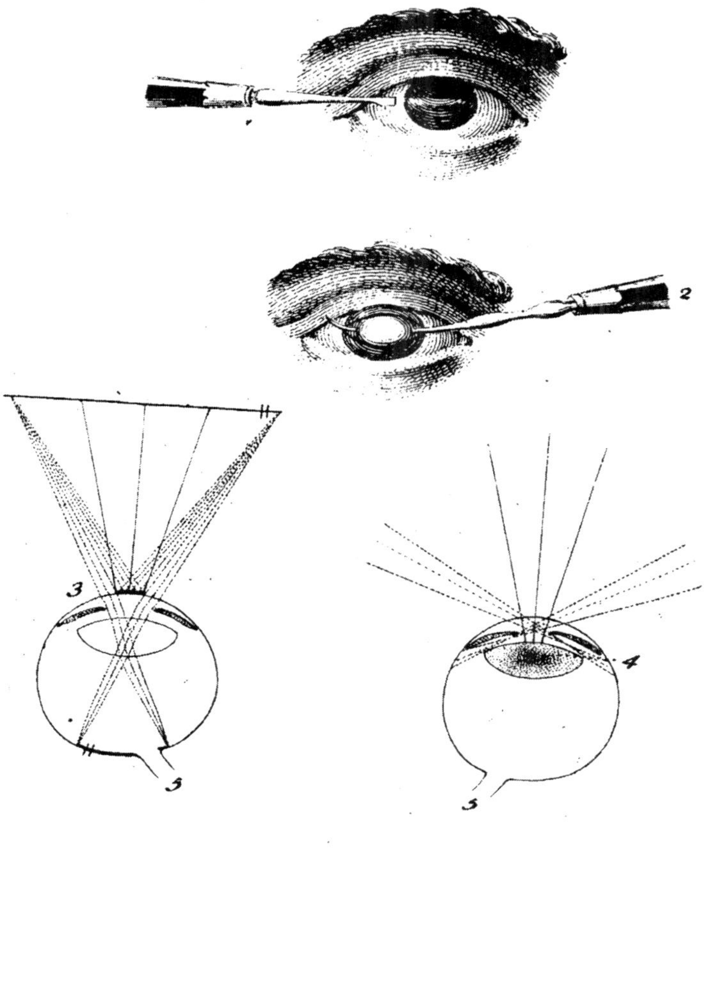

TAB. XXXVI.

1 A knife paſſed through the tunica ſclerotis, under the cornea before the iris, in order to cut an artificial pupil where the natural one is cloſed. This operation I have performed ſeveral times, with good ſucceſs; indeed it cannot fail when the operation is well done, and the eye no otherwiſe diſeaſed, which is more than can be ſaid for couching a cataract. In this operation great care muſt be taken to hold open the eyelids without preſſing upon the eye, for if the aqueous humour is ſqueezed out before the inciſion is made in the iris, the eye grows flaccid, and renders the operation difficult.

2 A crooked needle paſſed through a proptoſis of the cornea; the black line in the cornea incloſes the piece to be cut out with a knife. The operation being thus done, the cryſtalline humour immediately falls out; and in a few days the lips of the wound unite. This operation is very uſeful, and attended with but little pain. I have done the ſame thing when the whole eye has been ſo enlarged that the eyelids could not be cloſed, which has ſunk the eye in the head; but this operation was attended with ſuch violent pain that I cannot much recommend it.

3 Shews

3 Shews how an opake ſcar upon the cornea, by obſtructing part of each pencil of rays, makes a dimneſs of ſight without a total loſs.

4 Shews how a cataract or obſtruction of the cryſtalline humour, will obſtruct the light which is before it. And how ſome ſide-light may paſs to the retina through the aqueous humour, but not being brought into a focus gives only a ſenſe of light without viſion.

TAB. XXXVII.

TAB.XXXVII. P. 319.

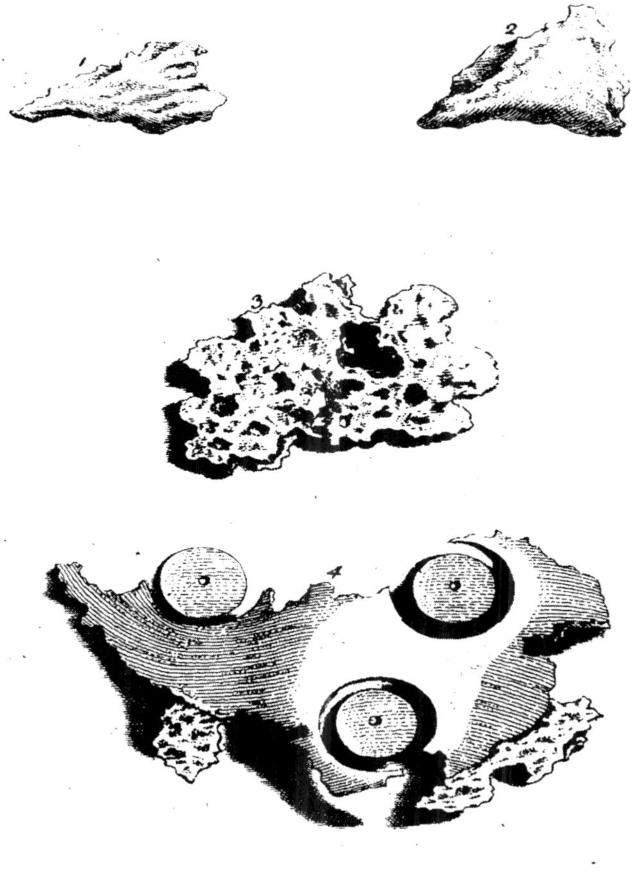

TAB. XXXVII.

1 A bone taken out from the firſt proceſs of the dura mater not far from the criſta galli.

2 A bone taken out of the muſcular part of the heart of a man.

3 The under ſide of a bone taken out of a fractured ſkull.

4 The upper ſide of a bone from the ſame ſkull, where the operation of the trepan had been thrice made. This girl was brought into the hoſpital a week after the accident. I immediately opened the ſcalp, and let out about two ounces of grumous blood, and laid the ſcull bare about four inches one way, and three the other, and tied the blood-veſſels, that I might make the operation without much difficulty ſoon after. The fracture extended acroſs the os bregmatis from the ſagittal ſuture to the temporal bone; that part next the os frontis was depreſſed equal to its thickneſs, and a great deal of extravaſated blood, and ſome matter lay under the other part of the ſame bone. I made two perforations with the trephine, cloſe to the fracture, that I might raiſe it up ſteddily through both, and have more room for the extravaſated blood to diſcharge from under the ſkull, which had diſcharged before in great quantity through the fracture. But never-

neverthelefs ten days after the former operation I was obliged to make another perforation to difcharge the matter more freely; for, during a month, the matter ran through all her dreffings down her face twice every day, and was exceedingly fetid, and for the fpace of three months the matter decreafed very little in quantity, but grew lefs and lefs offenfive. September the thirteenth, the leaft of the bones was taken out; and on September the twenty-ninth, the large one; after which time the matter was good, and not too much in quantity. Each of thefe bones is through both tables, for the motion in the brain was feen, only fome little parts of the leffer bone remaining, a callus was formed from them; but where the great one came away there was no callus, only a common cicatrix; and befides thefe, many little bits of bone came away in the dreffings: She was foon after cured, and has remained well many years.

T A B. XXXVIII.

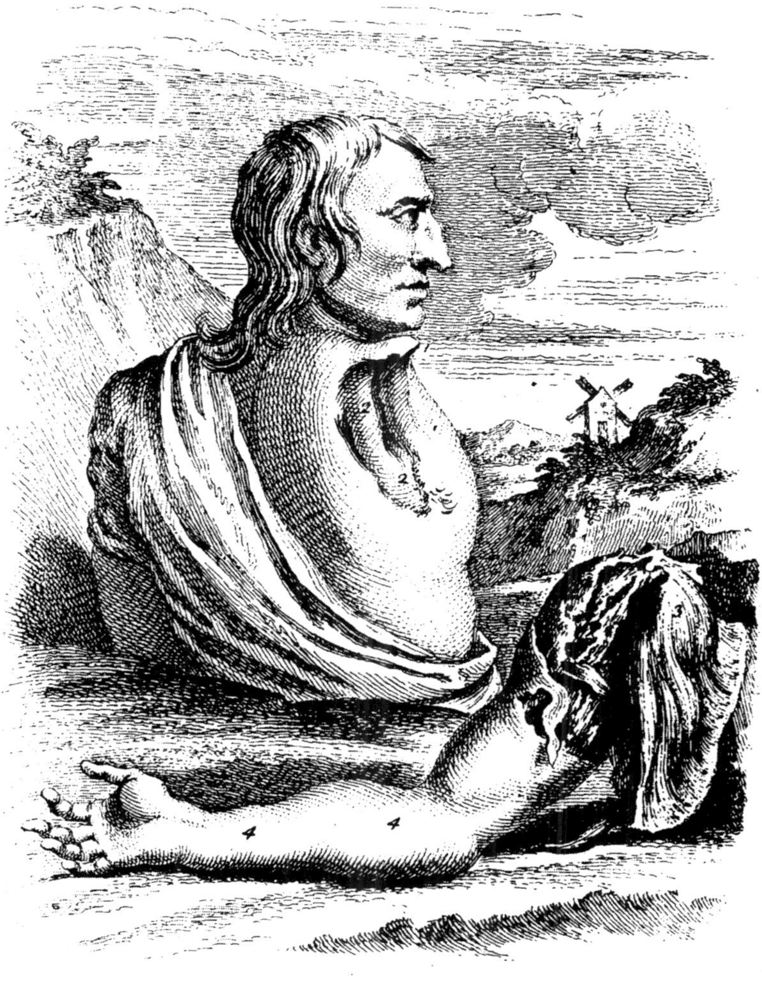
2
2
3
4
4

TAB. XXXVIII.

THE figure of SAMUEL WOOD, a miller, whoſe arm with the ſcapula was torn off from his body, by a rope winding round it, the other end being faſten'd to the coggs of a mill. This happen'd in the year 1737. The veſſels being thus ſtretch'd bled very little, the arteries and nerves were drawn out of the arm; the ſurgeon who was firſt call'd plac'd them within the wound, and dreſſed it ſuperficially. The next day he was put under Mr. FERNE's care, at St. Thomas's hoſpital, but he did not remove the dreſſings for ſome days: The patient had no ſevere ſymptoms, and the wound was cur'd by ſuperficial dreſſings only, the natural ſkin being left almoſt ſufficient to cover it; which ſhould in all caſes be done as much as may be: Above twenty years ſince I introduc'd the method of amputating, by firſt dividing the ſkin and membrana adipoſa, lower than the place where the operation was to be finiſh'd, the advantages of which are now ſufficiently known.

1 The end of the clavicle.
2 The cicatrix.
3 The ſubſcapularis muſcle.
4 The cubit broke in two places.

TAB. XXXIX.

REPRESENTS the caſe of JOHN HEYSHAM, who, the Friday before Eaſter, in the year 1721, by over-ſtraining himſelf at work, had a rupture of the inteſtines into the ſcrotum, which could by no means be reduced. He was brought into St. Thomas's hoſpital the Monday following, and I would have performed the operation immediately, but he refuſing to ſubmit, it was deferred till Tueſday morning, when he being willing, I performed the operation, and making a large wound in the bottom of the abdomen, the inteſtines were eaſily reduced, and near a quart of water was diſcharged out of the ſcrotum at the ſame time. There had been a rupture of the omentum before, which being united to the ſcrotum and ſpermatic veſſels, I paſſed a needle with a double ligature (as is expreſſed in the plate) under that part of the omentum that adhered, ſo as not to hurt the ſpermatic veſſels; then cutting out the needle, I tied one of the ſtrings over the upper part of the omentum, and the other over the lower, and then cut off as much of it as was in the way. My reaſon for tying in this manner was to ſecure the blood-veſſels, which, I think, could not be done ſo well with one ligature, becauſe of the large-

neſs

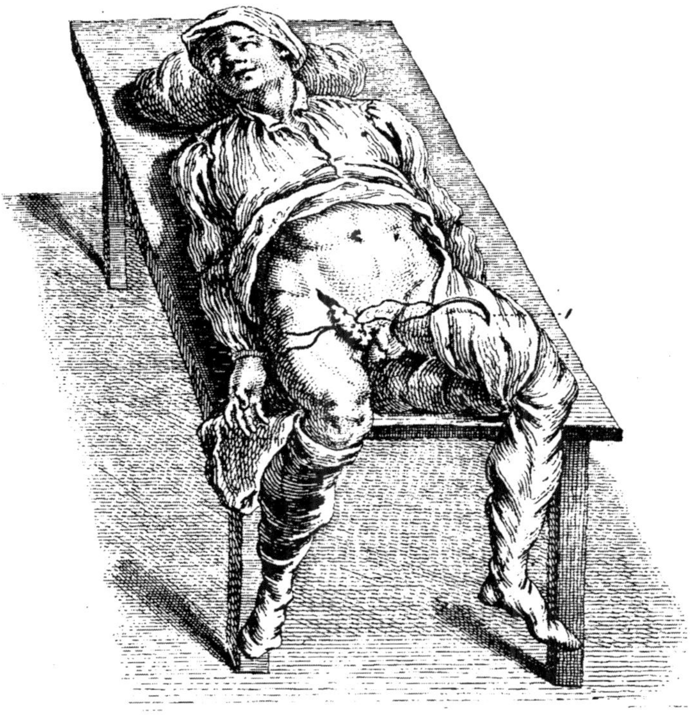

neſs of the adheſion and the texture of the omentum, which renders it too liable to be torn by ſuch a bandage. Three days after the operation an eryſipelas begun in his legs, and ſpread all over his body, the cuticle every where peeling off; yet he recovered, and continues in a good ſtate of health. After he was cured, at firſt he wore a ſmall truſs, but left it off in a ſhort time, and now feels no inconvenience from it, though he lives by hard labour.

TAB. XL.

The caſe of MARGARET WHITE, the wife of JOHN WHITE, a penſioner in the fiſhmongers alms-houſes at Newington in Surry. In the fiftieth year of her age, ſhe had a rupture at her navel, which continued till her ſeventy third year, when after a fit of the cholic, it mortified, and ſhe being preſently after taken with a vomiting, it burſt. I went to her and found her in this condition, with about ſix and twenty inches and an half of the gut hanging out, mortified. I took away what was mortified, and left the end of the ſound gut hanging out at the navel, to which it afterwards adhered; ſhe recovered, and lived many years after, voiding the excrements through the inteſtine at the navel; and though the ulcer was ſo large, after the mortification ſeparated, that the breadth of two guts was ſeen; yet they never at any time protruded out at the wound, though ſhe was taken out of her bed, and ſat up every day.

1 The gut.
2 The cicatrix of the wound.

CHAP.

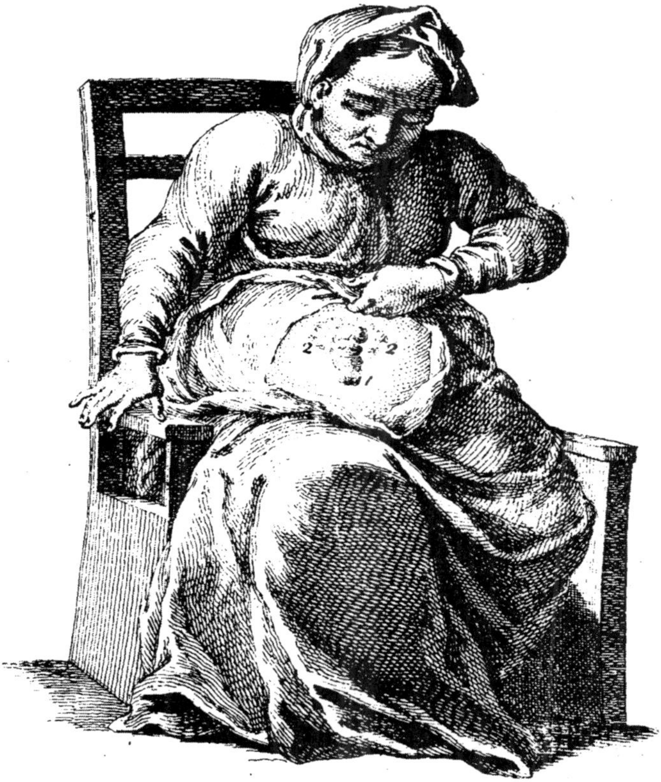
2
2
1

CHAPTER VI.

A ſhort hiſtorical account of cutting for the ſtone.

THE moſt ancient way of cutting for the ſtone is that deſcribed by CELSUS, which was indeed cutting upon the gripe, but in a very different manner from that operation in later ages, for he directs a lunated inciſion with the horns towards the coccyges, which was plainly that the gut might be preſſed downwards to avoid wounding it, and then a tranſverſe inciſion upon the ſtone might be made ſafely, but not in very young hildren, for want of room, nor after puberty, for then the proſtatæ are too large to allow of this operation; therefore they did not uſually cut any younger than nine years, nor older than fourteen: Afterwards, but when we know not, this operation was improved by cutting lower, and on one ſide, which is the operation now called cutting on the gripe, or with the leſſer apparatus.

IN the year 1524, MARIANUS publiſhed the method of cutting by the greater apparatus, now commonly call'd the old way, but he owns it was invented by his Maſter JOHANNES DE ROMANIS.

IN the year 1697, FRERE JACQUES came to Paris, full of reputation for the ſucceſs of his new operation for the ſtone; he ſoon obtain'd leave to cut in the hoſpitals, where great numbers of his patients dying, and being diſſected, they were found with their bladders cut through, guts wounded, &c. which brought the operation into diſgrace, as MERY and DIONIS have related, who ſaw theſe things. They ſay he performed the operation without any direction, and without any knowledge of the parts he was to cut; a thing not to be mentioned without horror! But of late his character has been ſet in a very different light; and though 'tis more than probable he himſelf knew not what he did, yet there are now, who pretend to tell us exactly, though if their teſtimonies are to be regarded, who ſaw him operate, there is no place that he did not cut one time or other, and therefore he may have a ſort of right to be call'd the inventor of any operation for the ſtone that can ever be performed in theſe parts. It is alſo own'd that he ſometimes had great ſucceſs, which was enough to put others of that nation upon trying of it in a more judicious manner; but if there were ſuch, failing of ſucceſs, they have conceal'd their experiments.

MR. RAU of Amſterdam, who ſaw F. JACQUES operate, profeſs'd to do his operation with the neceſſary improvement of a grooved ſtaff, which, if JACQUES ever uſed, he ſurely learned that of RAU. He ſucceeded wonderfully; and if he, who was an excellent anatomiſt, may be allow'd to underſtand his own operation, it was directly into the bladder, without wounding either the urethra

or

or the proſtates: beſides this, other competent judges, who were witneſſes to his operations, have bore the ſame teſtimony.

In the year 1717-18, Doctor James Douglass, in a paper preſented to the Royal Society, demonſtrated, from the anatomy of the parts, that the high operation for the ſtone might be practiſed; which had been once performed by Franco injudiciouſly, and by him diſrecommended, though his patient recovered; and afterwards ſtrongly recommended, but not practiſed by Rosset. Yet no one undertook it, till his brother Mr. John Douglass, about three years after, performed it, and with great applauſe, his two firſt patients recovering. Soon after, a ſurgeon of St. Thomas's hoſpital cut two, who both recovered; but the ſame gentleman afterwards cutting two, who miſcarried by the cutting or burſting the peritonæum, ſo that the guts appeared, this way immediately became as much decried as it was before commended; upon which the ſurgeons of St. Bartholomew's hoſpital, who had prepared to perform this operation, altered their reſolution, and went on in the old way. The next ſeaſon, it being my turn in St. Thomas's, I reſumed the high way, and cutting nine with ſucceſs, it came again in vogue; after that every lithotomiſt of both hoſpitals practiſed it; but the peritonæum being often cut or burſt, twice in my practice, though ſome of theſe recovered, and ſometimes the bladder itſelf was burſt, from injecting too much water, which generally proved fatal in a day or two. Another inconvenience attended every operation of this kind, which was, that the urine's lying continually in the wound, retarded the cure, but then it was never followed with an incontinence of urine. What the ſucceſs of the ſeveral operators was, I will not take the liberty to publiſh; but for my own, excluſive of the two before mentioned, I loſt no more than one in ſeven, which is more than any one elſe that I know of could ſay; whereas in the old way, even at Paris, from a fair calculation of above 800 patients, it appears that near two in five died. And though this operation came into univerſal diſcredit, I muſt declare it my opinion, that it is much better than the old way, to which they all returned, except myſelf, who would not have left the high way but for the hopes I had of a better; being well aſſured, that it might hereafter be practiſed with greater ſucceſs; theſe fatal accidents having pretty well ſhewn how much water might be injected, and how large the wound might ſafely be made. But hearing of the great ſucceſs of Mr. Rau, profeſſor of anatomy at Leyden, I determined to try, though not in his manner, to cut directly into the bladder; and as his operation was an improvement of Friar Jacques, I endeavoured to improve upon him, by filling the bladder, as Douglass had done in the high way, with water, leaving the catheter in, and then cutting on the outſide of the catheter into the bladder, in the ſame place as upon the gripe, which I could do very readily, and take out a ſtone of any ſize with more eaſe than in any other way. My patients for ſome days after the operation ſeemed out of danger; but the urine which came out of the bladder continually lodging upon the cellular membrane on the outſide of the rectum, made fœtid ulcers, attended with a vaſt diſcharge of ſtinking matter; and from this cauſe I loſt four patients out of ten. The caſe of one which eſcaped was very remarkable; a few days after he was cut, he was ſeized with a great pain in his back and legs, with very little power to move them; upon which he turned upon his face, and reſted almoſt conſtantly upon his knees and elbows above a fortnight together, having no eaſe in any other poſture all that while; at length his urine coming all the right way, his wound ſoon healed, and he recovered the uſe of his back and limbs. I think all theſe ſevere ſymptoms could proceed from no other cauſe than the urine and matter ſomehow offending the great nerves; which come out of the os ſacrum to go to the lower limbs. I then tried to cut into the bladder, in the ſame manner that Mr. Rau was commonly reported to do, but there had the ſame inconvenience from the urine's lodging upon the cellular membrane on the outſide of the inteſtinum rectum. Upon theſe diſap-

diſappointments, I contrived the manner of cutting, which is now called the lateral way. This operation I do in the following manner: I tie the patient as for the greater apparatus, but lay him upon a blanket ſeveral doubles upon an horizontal table three foot high, with his head only raiſed. I firſt make as long an inciſion as I can, beginning near the place where the old operation ends, and cutting down between the muſculus accelerator urinæ, and erector penis, and by the ſide of the inteſtinum rectum: I then feel for the ſtaff, holding down the gut all the while with one or two fingers of my left hand, and cut upon it in that part of the urethra which lies beyond the corpora cavernoſa urethræ, and in the proſtate gland, cutting from below upwards, to avoid wounding the gut; and then paſſing the gorget very carefully in the groove of the ſtaff into the bladder, bear the point of the gorget hard againſt the ſtaff, obſerving all the while that they do not ſeparate, and let the gorget ſlip to the outſide of the bladder; then I paſs the forceps into the right ſide of the bladder, the wound being on the left ſide of the perinæum; and as they paſs, carefully attend to their entering the bladder, which is known by their overcoming a ſtraitneſs which there will be in the place of the wound; then taking care to puſh them no further, that the bladder may not be hurt, I firſt feel for the ſtone with the end of them, which having felt, I open

I open the forceps and ſlide one blade underneath it, and the other at top; and if I apprehend the ſtone is not in the right place of the forceps, I ſhift it before I offer to extract, and then extract it very deliberately, that it may not ſlip ſuddenly out of the forceps, and that the parts of the wound may have time to ſtretch, taking great care not to gripe it ſo hard as to break it, and if I find the ſtone very large, I again cut upon it as it is held in the forceps. Here I muſt take notice, it is very convenient to have the bladder empty of urine before the operation, for if there is any quantity to flow out of the bladder at the paſſing in of the gorget, the bladder does not contract but collapſe into folds, which makes it difficult to lay hold of the ſtone without hurting the bladder; but if the bladder is contracted, it is ſo eaſy to lay hold of it, that I have never been delayed one moment, unleſs the ſtone was very ſmall. Laſtly, I tie the blood-veſſels by the help of a crooked needle, and uſe no other dreſſing than a little bit of lint beſmear'd with blood, that it may not ſtick too long in the wound, and all the dreſſings during the cure are very ſlight, almoſt ſuperficial, and without any bandage to retain them; becauſe that will be wetted with urine, and gall the ſkin. At firſt I keep the patient very cool to prevent bleeding, and ſometimes apply a rag dipt in cold water, to the wound, and to the genital parts, which I have found very uſeful in hot

weather

weather particularly. In children it is often alone ſufficient to ſtop the bleeding, and always helpful in men. The day before the operation I give a purge to empty the guts, and never neglect to give ſome laxative medicine or clyſter a few days after, if the belly is at all tenſe, or if they have not a natural ſtool. What moved me to try this way, if I may be allowed to know my own thoughts, was the conſideration of women ſcarce ever dying of this operation; from which I concluded, that if I could cut into the urethra, beyond the corpora cavernoſa urethræ, the operation would be nearly as ſafe in men as women.

WHAT ſucceſs I have had in my private practice I have kept no account of, becauſe I had no intention to publiſh it, that not being ſufficiently witneſſed. Publickly in St. Thomas's hoſpital I have cut two hundred and thirteen; of the firſt fifty only three died; of the ſecond fifty, three; of the third fifty, eight; and of the laſt ſixty-three, ſix. Several of theſe patients had the ſmall pox during their cure, ſome of which died, but I think not more in proportion than what uſually die of that diſtemper; theſe are not reckon'd among thoſe who died of the operation. The reaſon why ſo few died in the two firſt fifties was, at that time few very bad caſes offer'd; in the third, the operation being in high requeſt, even the moſt aged and moſt miſerable caſes expected to be ſav'd by it; beſides, at that time, I made the operation lower

lower in hopes of improving it, but found I was miſtaken. But what is of moſt conſequence to be known is the ages of thoſe who recovered, and thoſe who died. Of theſe, under ten years of age one hundred and five were cut, three died; between ten and twenty, ſixty-two cut, four died; twenty and thirty, twelve cut, three died; thirty and forty, ten cut, two died; forty and fifty, ten cut, two died; fifty and ſixty, ſeven cut, four died; ſixty and ſeventy, five cut, one died; between ſeventy and eighty, two cut, one died. Of thoſe who recovered the three biggeſt ſtones were ℥ xii, x¼, and viii, and the greateſt number of ſtones in any one perſon was thirty three. One of the three that died out of the hundred and five, was very ill with a whooping cough; another bled to death by an artery into the bladder, it being very hot weather at that time: But this accident taught me afterwards, whenever a veſſel bled that I could not find, to dilate the wound with a knife, till I could ſee it. Now if JACQUES or others, who of late have been ſaid to have performed this operation, whether by deſign or chance, did not take care to ſecure the blood-veſſels, which as yet has not been ſuppoſed, whatever their dexterity in operating might be, their ſucceſs at leaſt can be no ſecret, for many of their children and moſt of their men patients muſt have bled to death. If I have any reputation in this way,

I have

I have earn'd it dearly, for no one ever endured more anxiety and ſickneſs before an operation, yet from the time I began to operate, all uneaſineſs ceaſed; and if I have had better ſucceſs than ſome others, I do not impute it to more knowledge, but to the happineſs of a mind that was never ruffled or diſconcerted, and a hand that never trembled during any operation.

INDEX.

INDEX.

Artery,

INDEX.

Bones,

Dentes.

I N D E X.

Figures

INDEX.

Gland,

Os

Processus

Skin

FINIS.